·Spare Days·

Also by Marvin Barrett
The Jazz Age
The Years Between
The End of the Party

Du Pont Columbia Surveys
Broadcast Journalism
The Eye of the Storm (with Zachary Sklar)
Rich News, Poor News
Moments of Truth?
The Politics of Broadcasting
State of Siege
Year of Challenge, Year of Crisis
Survey of Broadcast Journalism 1968–1969

·Spare Days·

Marvin Barrett

Arbor House · William Morrow
New York

818.54
BaR

882890

Library of Congress Cataloging-in-Publication Data

Barrett, Marvin.
Spare days / by Marvin Barrett. — 1st ed.
p. cm.
ISBN 1-557-10006-3 : $17.95
1. Barrett, Marvin—Diaries. 2. Authors, American—20th century—
Diaries. 3. Cancer—Patients—United States—Diaries. 4. Heart—
Diseases—Patients—United States—Diaries.   I. Title.
PS3552.A7347Z463 1987
818'.5403—dc19
[B]   87-33329   CIP

Printed in the United States of America

First Edition

1 2 3 4 5 6 7 8 9 10

To Mary Ellin

·Spare Days·

Preface

I was sixty-three when I began this journal. I know nothing magical about the number 63, but in my life, as the following pages bear witness, that year brought a crisis—physical, mental, spiritual—of major proportions. Not that the three aspects were separable, although at the beginning of this account I was still stubbornly trying to separate them.

To be more specific: (1) I was under treatment for bleeding ulcers—four Tagaments a day in addition to the three Cardizems I had been taking faithfully to compensate for a myocardial infarction suffered four years earlier. (2) The bleeding ulcers suggested that the low-grade depression I had been experiencing might deserve professional attention. A pleasant young Freudian analyst was enlisted to hear my ill-defined complaints once a week. (3) Undergirding my queasy stomach, heavy heart, and light head, exacerbating and alleviating them by turns, was a spiritual struggle, a one-man soap opera, which had been going on for well over forty years. Nothing new there. A sometime member of a Gurdjieff group that met every Thursday evening to explore ways of spiritual growth, also a practicing Episcopalian, I had taken daily rather than weekly communion during the previous Advent, attended to my Lenten duties, added devotional reading to the morning prayers I faithfully pursued—thirty minutes before my morning walk and breakfast—all to no apparent avail. Things were getting more scrambled by the hour.

Professionally it seemed to me that I was in trouble. The people who had paid my salary for the past fifteen years, trustees of a foundation that second-guessed my decisions from a skyscraper a thousand miles to the south of Columbia University, my place of work, appeared disenchanted with me. When I had a success, they chose to ignore it. Their suggestions for improvement were insensitive and ill-informed.

My thirty-one-year marriage, it seemed to me, had seen better days. I felt myself boring and yet ill-used. My children and my wife were both a comfort and a concern, depending upon my mood, which was increasingly glum.

In my jaundiced view I had been surer, steadier at a third my present age, when, on the lip of World War II, Aldous Huxley and Gerald Heard had signed me up for Trabuco, their religious commune in the hills of Southern California. A few months later I was swept off to naval service on the shores of the Coral Sea. No matter. I prayed six hours a day under the swaying palms. Convinced and devout, I knew life's meaning and my purpose on earth; exactly where I was heading and what I should do to get there. Whatever bloody battles were going on in the Solomons to the north or on the other side of the globe simply reinforced my convictions.

Nor had I ever completely relinquished that suspicion that life's meaning was accessible to all men and women of good will, and yet forty years later, I was a mess. A privileged mess, to be sure, with an apartment in town, a house in the country, a beautiful and clever wife, four splendid children. At this juncture, circumstances, one circumstance in particular, persuaded me that I should keep a diary. This is something, though I have been committed to words as my living since I was twenty-seven, I have never had the wits nor energy to stick with for more than a self-conscious day or two. This journal went on for over seven months.

The following excerpts seem to me the most coherent passages—the ones that best give the picture of a man, certainly no better and probably not much worse than most, who narrowly escaped bad trouble, or at least learned to redefine what bad trouble might be.

Conceivably anyone who has shared a portion of that trouble and the comfort it called forth may find something familiar and of use in what I have put down of my own experience.

At any rate, here it is.

I.

Morningside Heights, Manhattan

September

1. The call came yesterday evening during dinner. I took it on the kitchen phone with the swinging door open so that the doctor's message—"Mr. Barrett, I am afraid you have cancer," no beating about the bush, flat out in her pleasant, dry drawl—must have been obvious to anyone who heard my end of the conversation. "I thought you'd prefer to find out about it at home rather than in the office," Dr. W. said with a hint of apology before she rang off. I confirmed the news when I rejoined Mary Ellin and Irving at the table.

There was no immediate emotional display from my wife and son, nor did I feel the lack of one. For some reason, I experienced no particular shock at being given, without preparation, what many of us might consider the ultimate bad news. I had been much more shocked when, sitting on the sofa in the living room window some months earlier, M., an old and dear friend of ours, told me she had cancer. And it wasn't because that was a surprise. The signs of her struggle, if you wished to read them, had been on her for months—the loss of weight, the hair suddenly cropped, the pallor, the languor, the too bright eyes—though the symptoms were always given alter-

nate readings so that if you loved her and saw her only inter-
mittently you need not have acknowledged the truth. And yet
the suspicion lay there all the more potent for being resisted,
for being unconfirmed. How potent was apparent when she
made her confession. It was such a cry: not loud, not defiant,
but sharp, nonetheless, right to the gut. She cared. That simple
statement, "Marvin, I've got cancer"—the voice breaking, the
tears not spilling, but standing there in her eyes—said that she
wanted to live, that she wasn't sure she would, and that what
I'd known all along was suddenly the unbearable truth. Now
I had my own truth to convey.

But the information that Dr. W. gave me, which I passed
along to Mary Ellin and Irving—that there was indication of
a malignancy, that surgery might be required, had none of that
horror, that disbelief and pain. My response was to sit down
and finish what was left on my plate. The Depression child
doing his duty. "Marvin, eat your macaroni and cheese."
"Marvin, eat your chipped beef. Would you rather have bread
and milk?" Tonight it was chicken and string beans.

Mary Ellin came over and hugged me, brushing her
dark hair against my cheek. Irving, a tall, blond, thoughtful
twenty-eight-year-old, said little or nothing. What, after all,
was there to say? Eventually he cleared away the plates,
stacked the dishes in the dishwasher, and, wiping his hands
on his paint-spattered khakis, went back to his drawing
board. Mary Ellin and I sat in silence. Not stunned silence.
Just silence.

How could I have cancer? I was a heart patient. Members
of my family were all heart patients. Cancer was not our way.
Our way was sudden, not slow death.

After sitting there at the empty table for a while, Mary

Ellin and I went out for a walk along Claremont Avenue, up 116th Street, and down Broadway to Baskin and Robbins, where I had my first ice cream cone in over four years.

IT had been four years and two months since that day in July when, the perfect candidate for a coronary—overweight, tense, meeting deadlines—I finally lived up to everyone's expectations. I had my heart attack while eating a pear and cottage cheese salad in the same kitchen where I received Dr. W.'s call. Irving, who happened to be in the apartment, phoned the doctor, two doctors (one was in Beirut, the other out to lunch), a hospital (no ambulances available), the police (they'd look into it). Finally, an hour and a half later, two young men in fatigues came into the back bedroom, gave me a skeptical once over, took my blood pressure and pulse, and reluctantly led me away.

I had behaved myself perfectly ever since, losing weight, taking long, brisk walks every morning, watching my liquor, carrying my bottle of nitroglycerine tablets, sticking meticulously to a low-cholesterol diet—no eggs, no bacon, no butter, no ice cream, no chocolate. Now I was eating a pistachio, almond fudge double-dip cone. There has been no diet prescribed for cancer . . . yet.

And where in God's name did the cancer come from? How long have I been working on it? Since last Thanksgiving when, without occasion or explanation the bottom seemed to fall out of everything and I took to attending 7:15 communion at St. John the Divine every morning just to get from one day to the next? Or was it earlier than that, in Aspen, when I was having my hiatus hernia that turned out to be appendicitis? Or earlier even than that—built into my life, inherent, as my brother's first wife used to say, in the germ plasm?

Or does my cancer have something to do with where I live: 35 Claremont Avenue. Four neighbors on the three floors below me, all dead of cancer in half a decade. And now, coming up to the fourth floor, me. It never occurred to me that I might be next.

And I really don't know yet exactly what I have—how big, how malignant, exactly where it is. "We think we've found it early. It is a small area," said Dr. W. But how early is early? And how small is small?

For the past several years I have been trying to pray below the head, across my chest, as though my arms were the bar of a cross, and that, more or less, is where, I guess, the cancer must be.

THURSDAY morning, twelve hours before Dr. W.'s call, I was told I seemed troubled at the service in the cathedral and at breakfast after. I was, I admit, wound tight, apprehensive, as I have been throughout so much of my life—not about Wednesday's test or the results, which I had completely forgotten, but about everything, about nothing—and feeling guilt in the presence of the dean and his wife. Ever cheerful, cheering the rest of us on, they had just been through the ordeal of a desperately sick daughter, enduring a horrendous operation for Hodgkins disease—a tissue of dead cells lying across her lungs, casting a sinister, inexplicable shadow, which once discovered had to be pulled off like the film from a rice pudding, the scum from a brackish pond. I seemed troubled!

Then back to the Journalism School, to my office where

videocassette after videocassette of documentaries dealing with other people's troubles, most of them insoluble, were waiting to be watched, part of my job as Director of the DuPont Columbia Awards in Broadcast Journalism, evaluating other people's tapes, other people's troubles. I treated myself to four of the most depressing: on child abuse, on Alzheimer's disease, on the Cuban criminals from Mariel, on child suicide.

After lunch I got a call from Mr. D., the eighty-six-year-old I visit weekly—holed up, alone, and ailing in an Upper West Side hotel. Now, Mr. D., an ex cashier, floorwalker, singer, hoofer, M.C. radio star, bartender, a sometime buddy of Imogene "Bubbles" Wilson and Kiki Roberts, with an iron constitution and erratic spirits, was summoning me to confer with him about his terminal arrangements, will, cremation, burial et al. He really didn't want to go on living. He had nothing to live for. And for the moment I had no argument to give him. As I listened, that precariousness and fear of not being able to find an answer, to cope, washed over me. Long before supper and the call from Dr. W.

SO today I told Oz Elliott Dr. W.'s news and enlisted him, as my superior officer, to take my place at the Radio and Television News Directors Convention in Las Vegas, where I was scheduled to make a few remarks. With his usual good humor he agreed, although it meant twenty-four sleepless hours in the murky splendors of Caesar's Palace—Cleopatra's Barge, the Circus Maximus, the clanking limbo between the elevator bank and the main desk, a limbo within a limbo. Me, saved by the knife.

2. Now, all at once, I find myself on two, not just one, heavily traveled paths to death. Not that death was much on my mind after my heart attack. Although there had been several sudden heart deaths in my family, Father had survived his first coronary and three more attacks for nearly thirty years. He finally slipped away in his sleep, without warning, a continent away, never, I was told, even stirring the covers.

In a moment, with half a dozen words, my defenses have been penetrated and the thought of death is right there, beside me.

And, thinking of death, I begin to consider not eternity, not oblivion, but what an intensely interesting life I've led. Not pleasant, necessarily, although there have been long pleasant stretches, but always interesting, even when it wasn't pleasant, particularly when it wasn't pleasant. Its surfaces have not been all that unusual: a would-be novelist turned journalist and editor, and then for the last fifteen years an academic grunt with a fancy title; a genius, like thousands of others, converted to householder and breadwinner. Still, since 1942, when Aldous Huxley and Gerald Heard converted me from Ivy League skepticism to post-Bloomsbury piety, I have been engaged, with varying degrees of concentration in a search to find meaning in life's detail as well as its large dispositions, observing, sometimes bleakly, sometimes with delighted wonder, what was going on around me and inside me, occasionally attempting to change what I saw. And if such a search contributed pain, fear, stress, frustration, a dozen other discomforts to life's unfolding, it also added unfailing interest. And there are the further ranges of meaning that Mary Ellin's and the children's lives, intertwined with mine, suggest. And all those beyond. At sixty-three the process goes on, disquieting, fascinating.

Central to the search, always there, is prayer. The fact of it, its possibilities. The bland, innocuous word, the towering reality. I can't claim my practice of it is in any way expert, but I am grateful to know that the activity exists to be pursued, however distractedly. There it is, for me, a room next to, if not a doorway into reality. And there is always the hope that by stubbornness or grace, or a combination of the two, I will get through, break into the place beyond. Me . . . there, at the source of all strength and transformation.

MEANWHILE, some questions.

How long have I had it? Where did it come from?

Why me? Not: Why me and not somebody else? But what did I do, think, eat, invite into me to bring this about?

And how will I use it? Am I already using it? To feel more, less guilty? To get sympathy? To make others feel guilty? To get out of things I would otherwise have felt obliged to do? What does it do really to my sense of time—to the past, the future, right now? Is that sense sharpened, or blurred, or perhaps both? Do I really see life more clearly now than two days ago? Will I do different things or the same things differently? Will I become more independent? More dependent? How will I avoid becoming a thing—that rapture of the hospital—being wheeled about at six thousand dollars a day? All that funny money paying for big contraptions, big procedures, a whole new set of procedures.

Cancer will be different.

3. When all this began last July with those inconsequential symptoms—faintness, nausea—it was assumed that my heart, despite my exemplary behavior, was acting up. A dizzy spell while waiting for the seventh-floor elevator at the Journalism School after a day of watching tapes of TV documentaries, attempting to judge the unjudgeable—to say what is good and what is bad, honoring the good with an Alfred I. Du Pont Columbia University Award in Broadcast Journalism, a silver baton with the winner's name on it. Good! Hour after hour of intolerable, insoluble problems: mental hospitals, nursing homes, prisons, incurable diseases, ecological disasters, technological failures, war, famine, plague, scams, shakedowns, stakeouts. Fifteen years I had been watching them—the same shows, the same problems and catastrophes never getting any better. Why shouldn't I feel dizzy?

I went back to my desk to wait for the spell to pass. When it didn't I put in a call to my cardiologist, Dr. Miles Schwartz. He ordered me across campus to St. Luke's.

There was a puzzled two-day stopover in intensive care, me with my red beach face sitting up reading my *New York Times,* my trendy books in their bright jackets, cracking jokes with the nurses when all about me were prone bodies, motionless and speechless, plugged into a dozen gurgling, bleeping machines, being lived by their machines.

Then on to cardiac care and the tests—putting me on bicycles, on treadmills, making me trudge, pedal up make-believe hills, threading wires from my groin up some vein or artery into my heart, flushing it with dye, a rush of warmth; none of this seemed particularly relevant or really necessary. The heart was fine. Then, at the last minute, the real culprit, unmasked by some minor check: a stomach ulcer, bleeding. Hence the nausea, the faintness—humiliating, not threatening. All that time and trouble for a mingy little ulcer. Two months worth of pills, four a day, and a tube stuck down my throat to make sure all was well.

And now, thanks to that tube and a few bits of tissue clipped from my stomach, they tell me that in a week or so I'll be back in the hospital. More tests. A lot more tests and then surgery.

WHY do I, all at once, believe this is serious, serious in a way that what has gone before has never been? Here is something that has to be confronted and coped with, that can't be ignored or avoided. Just because it is cancer.

Water Mill, Long Island

1. I went to church for the first time since I got the news—St John's in Southampton, the Sunday 9:30 A.M. service. I found myself listening harder than usual, although I am not a particularly inattentive member of the congregation. I have always looked for messages that speak to my condition, over the others' heads. A questionable practice—like looking for the almonds in a bowl of mixed nuts, the chocolates with a hard center. There were a few. Verse five of the processional hymn, "Coronation."

> Sinners, who love can ne'er forget
> The wormwood and the gall,
> Go spread your trophies at his feet,
> And crown him lord of all!

Gall: "a tumor caused by irritation, anything bitter or distasteful, impudence, brazen assurance." Wormwood: "any unpleasant or mortifying experience"—trophies for spreading.

The gospel was Luke 15:1–10, the parable of the lost sheep. A little gentler, more reassuring. Maybe.

And finally the recessional, unfamiliar words and tune, and I was back out in the hot bright September morning, having told no one, no one the wiser.

There were hot bright mornings at Trabuco as well, an endless sequence of them, and secrets not told. Trabuco, it floated up before me like a mirage, the long white walls, the pink roof, the belfry with its verdigrised bell, a convent from the Balearic Isles slung in the saddle of a Southern California hill, halfway between the mountains and the sea, where the search for meaning could be begun under the optimum conditions. A kind of paradise, or so it seemed to me at first forty years ago.

The oratory. The hymn we sang in it. New words set to a Bach chorale

> The lord of life has called us.
> Why stand we idle here?
> Have grief and pain appalled us?
> Is empty death our fear?

With perfect clarity the sound and the scene returned to me: the dozen voices in the damp, cold oratory with its smell of new plaster; the rough carpet, Another smell; the steps down into the octagonal pit, dark with only the reflection of yesterday's sun on the cruxorata against the far wall. And after the prayers, two hours of them, coming back out into the hot morning sun on the porch where we put on our shoes and headed up the broad shallow steps through the cloisters, past the library to the refectory, where Gerald Heard, our leader and teacher, although he denied his worthiness to be either, read to us from Father Faber, the Venerable Augustine Baker, Patanjali, The Cloud of Unknowing, Milarepa, while we ate.

What would the fifty-eight-year-old Gerald make of me—a white-haired man with cancer, five years older than he was when I walked out on him and the others, when I fled in terror.

SO the speculations return. Why couldn't I, before I die, if indeed that is what they are telling me—that death will be sooner rather than later—why couldn't I dedicate my disease, whatever suffering it may entail, to some particular thing— homes for the homeless; world peace; help for delinquent boys, the needy, the old; a cure for cancer after I've gone? Offer it all up in exchange for a solution to at least one of those problems I have been staring at day after day, year after year. Not the silver baton (our equivalent of an Oscar) but, just for once, a solution.

But here I am, contemplating squandering on earth at the last minute what little treasure I may store up in the hereafter, a spendthrift to the end.

Waste, as Gerald would say, is the sin against the holy ghost. There was, in his philosophy, more than one such sin.

I begin to think about the other deaths—not mine, but Mother's, Father's, Eddie's. Not my reaction to the deaths, but the quality of the deaths themselves—whether they made "good" deaths. What is a "good" death for a three-year-old? How does it differ from a sixty-year-old's death. And why do I think that, if I can behave myself, for me at least, a death with a warning that I take seriously, that I can prepare for, is to be preferred? Mother, all over in a matter of hours. Poppa, a dozen warnings, then going in his sleep. Eddie, the three-year-old, the baby, suddenly, violently struck down at the top of the hill—the Avenue that we had been warned against time and again: "Stop. Look both ways . . ."—with me, his eight-year-old brother, standing on the curb, my hand, which had held his, empty, grasping nothing. The gray Essex sedan, the instrument of death, coming to a screeching halt. Mother at home making dinner. Father due back any minute from work. Brother Dirk in the vacant lot playing ball. The aunts and uncles, the cousins, the grandparents, a town full of oblivious relatives and friends. And me with this horror in front of me, the small lifeless body, inescapably forever mine. The innocent. The guilty. I heard my voice. The wail. And looking neither way I ran down the hill past the car, the body, the cluster of anguished, ineffectual grownups. Ran home to 1408 Forestdale, the pretty little house beyond the hickory trees, four rooms and an attic, four wooden pillars across the open brick porch. The swing at one end. Motionless. A hot, clear, Iowa summer afternoon. July 2, 1928.

It was that afternoon, Gerald said, that drew me to religion, made it inevitable that at twenty-two I should dedicate my life to God. Nothing short of that dedication, Gerald said, could set that afternoon right.

2. I am, for the moment, for some mysterious reason, free from the anxiety that has been there for years. It is the period after the exams and before the grades, although it isn't really—the exams go on to the end—but there does seem, for the moment, a space, a let up.

Why should being reminded of the possibility of death

ten weeks or ten years away relieve me of anxiety, even temporarily? The certainty of death is a given—a constant in human life—yet being reminded of it lifts my most persistent pain, makes it possible for me to look at anything, almost anything. There is a magic apparently in the words "Cancer. I've got it."

3. Tonight we went to the movies in Easthampton to see *The Grey Fox,* a film with its aging scamps that evoked the generation before mine and the one before that— Uncle Leonard, great Uncle Marius, the old West. Uncle Leonard in the upstairs bedroom at Grandmother's house in San Diego with his six-shooter, his chaps, his lariat and ten-gallon hat, his coffin nails rolled with one hand, pulling the bag of Bull Durham closed with his teeth, a trick learned in Montana punching cattle. Uncle Marius in the Klondike with the mud black and thick as fudge, hip deep, and the mosquitoes as big as humming birds, a young man seeking his fortune— now a straight-backed eighty-year-old walking the five miles to Grandmother's house, rain or shine, without a pause. I recognize them, those aging men—failed perhaps, perhaps not (How could one gauge?)—certainly by now long dead and gone. Everyone, I suppose, has such men and women back there somewhere, larger than life, or maybe just magnified by time and distance.

There must be, even in the Hamptons, a few ne'er-do-wells and buccaneers telling their tall tales to goggle-eyed nephews and nieces. Fortunes lost, fame barely missed. But nothing stored up today can compare.

4. Now I have self-observation compounded. Not this diary, but my moment-by-moment attention to my stomach, the center, and to every little pang from foot to head that moves through my body. What does that mean—this twinge, that ache? Is that it? Has the crab crawled down—up—there? It is not panic, just curiosity. In a week or so I may know exactly. Be able to put everything in its place. Except I don't really want to know. A sort of cautious indifference protects me.

THIS morning, I woke up early. The train heading out to Montauk through the potato fields, or some noise in an old house full of unexplained noises had roused me. Thank God it was not Gerard Manley Hopkins's awful waking to "feel the fell of dark, not day" which I have had on and off for so many years, the three to six A.M. examen of everything about me and my life—inadvertently, then intentionally negative, piling it on just to see how much I can take, threat upon threat, failure upon failure, to prove to myself that it takes more than I know to obliterate hope. That exercise in defiance, piling up the shit three or four mornings a week, "a low-grade depression, clinically insignificant," then leaning into it with any prayer I could muster—"Almighty God. Almighty God. Have mercy upon me a miserable sinner." Holding it there, keeping it from falling, sliding over, inundating me; ceasing at dawn, out here when the birds begin, in New York when the bars on the bedroom ceiling cast by the light in the areaway finally fade away. Could all those mornings have brought me to this? Was that where the cancer came from?

* * *

A game . . . How will I spend my time—if I have any, that is, disposable, that is?

A month in the old hotel on the rim of the Grand Canyon? Darjeeling, Kanchenjunga from the veranda of the Windamere, perhaps a glimpse of Everest? The lowest, the highest visible places on earth.

A month at Trabuco with the Ramakrishna monks who have kept the place going now for nearly forty years since we all decamped?

Going back to Sicily? Our honeymoon revisited—Siracusa, Noto, Segesta, Cefalù, Agrigento.

The New Hebrides? Steaming into Port Vila, taking the washboard road across Efate through the banyan forests to Havannah Harbor and on to Quoin Hill. Seeing if it is the way I remember it: the water, chocolate brown and turquoise and across it the double volcano with its rose and green flanks.

Visiting Ceylon, Bali, New Zealand, Kyoto, Samoa, the places I've wanted to see and never have?

The Holy Land?

There are a lot of things one could do with a little time.

A tour of France with Irving, the artist.

A visit in San Francisco with Elizabeth, the teacher and young matron.

Maybe England with Mary Ellin Jr., the journalist.

Italy with Katherine, the scholar, who is already there.

Any or all of the above with M.E., depending on her whim.

And meanwhile, what happens to this farmhouse on Scuttle Hole Road, the dog I have yet to buy, the book that isn't yet written?

* * *

ELIZABETH and M.E. on the telephone discussing Henrietta, the little black cat—her accident in town, out the fourth floor window into the areaway, her broken leg. Four hundred dollars to have it set. How high would we have been willing to go was the question. For a stray cat. Five hundred dollars? One thousand dollars?

"How high would you be willing to go for a human being?" I ask M.E. when she finally rings off. "A hundred thousand dollars? Five hundred thousand dollars?"

"Oh, for you," M.E. says, "a million. Of course, unlike Henrietta, you have insurance."

5. Five A.M. Another early waking, thinking of Aldous Huxley. Aldous, Gerald's most famous convert, dying of cancer, doing his last assignment for me, his old high school fan, his disciple at one remove, now editor of a magazine rich enough to pay him well, dictating his last paragraphs from his death bed. "Shakespeare and Religion," but really about Shakespeare and death. Aldous citing those terrible lines from *Measure for Measure:*

Ay, but to die, and go we know not where;
To lie in cold obstruction, and to rot;

And then another, equally bleak passage, from *Macbeth.* And finally, Aldous, that master ventriloquist, having Shakespeare proclaim for him, via Prospero, the doctrine of Maya: "The world is an illusion, but it is an illusion which we must take seriously, because it is real as far as it goes, and in those aspects of the reality which we are capable of apprehending. Our business is to wake up." Aldous preaching to the very end. Dictating the gospel to his wife from his pillow. The next day he was dead.

I have obviously crossed a barrier, joined a crowd of witnesses that some time in the past commanded my awe, my love, my pity and dread.

Tilly Losch, Aldous's friend and mine. He knew her in her prime, the beautiful dancing girl from the corps de ballet of the Vienna Opera pretending to be a countess, succeeding. The toast of London—the nun in Max Reinhardt's *The Miracle* turned sinner then back to nun again. Tilly spinning through *Wake Up and Dream,* alongside the Astaires in *The Band Wagon,* with Lotte Lenya in *The Seven Deadly Sins,* on to Hollywood to be Paul Muni's exotic second wife in *The Good Earth*—my first view of her, me a mesmerized sixteen-year-old looking up at the silver screen in Des Moines's best picture palace, Tilly bigger than life, clearer.

Mary Ellin's and my Tilly was different, the kibitzer and standard-setter, the friend of the family. Tough, tender Tilly, in her cluttered Manhattan apartment with the mementos of her glamorous past, her mysterious, busy present, her jewels, her couturier clothes, hanging on, then fighting for every slipping inch, for her life, the effort turning her from a persistent, sloe-eyed thirties beauty into an ancient Chinese crone, sitting there in her hospital bed, her dancer's back straight until she died—her cancer finally winning—sitting up.

All the gang at 35 Claremont Avenue, floor by floor: Lionel Trilling, Prof. Ausubel, Dick Baker, Janet Kimball. Janet standing on the island on Broadway, big, pretty, in no way obviously dying, carrying a large flat paper parcel, her x-rays, no doubt her death warrant, jauntily under her arm. A few weeks later, gone.

And those others, I didn't know, that I watched to earn my living, live-on-tape, dying, then dead, flickering away on the screen across from me in my deep leather chair, behind me the pigeons cooing on the sill. There they were on the glass square, all those at-first hearty, gradually thinning, paling men and women, their cheerfulness slowly muting, stunned: the woman in Ohio, mother of seven, in her new wig, hope defined, and then slowly abandoned; the magazine editor, young, childless, two heart-breakingly bleak years in two and a half gruelling hours, her final almost senseless protests in the dark hospital room, the defeated doctor, the absent husband back too late, all on camera. An award winner—a silver baton. The army sergeant, present at the deadly tests in the desert, down wind from St. George, Utah, going from hale, handsome forty-year-old to a wasted, blotched, hairless skeleton, still capable of indignation, of speech, denouncing the government which he had served that could do this to him and then turn its back. Another silver baton.

Ah, but stop it . . . What makes me think I am one of them? They tell me they have found it early, that my chances are very good.

AFTER lunch, the beach. At Flying Point I suggest to a bunch of jocks, aged twelve to fifty, who have decided to play touch football where I have set up my chair that they might do better farther down the sand, and, wonder of wonders, they move on without rancor or insult. Nor do I feel the kind of petulance,

---

the sour guilt at spoiling someone else's fun that would have possessed me at an earlier date. Cancer seems to promote authority. Here is an old fellow beyond trifling with.

STILL, for long stretches today, I forgot the fate which, I suppose, could be said to hang over me. I don't know whether that might be considered a blessing or not.

Morningside Heights

1. I went to the 7:15 A.M. Thursday service at the cathedral—huge, dark, cool—a few of us in our chapel behind the high altar. I read the lesson from Isaiah: "But men will say to you, 'Seek guidance of ghosts and familiar spirits who squeak and gibber; a nation may surely seek guidance of its gods, of the dead on behalf of the living, for an oracle or a message.' They will surely say some such thing as this; but what they say is futile." I read loud. Then came the Beatitudes. Their simple unequivocal demands that one be poor in spirit, meek, pure in heart have always seemed too much for me. The Lord's Prayer is more appropriate to my condition.

After service, in the ambulatory Jim Morton, the man responsible for maintaining the largest church almost in Christendom, keeping the floor swept, the lamps lit, the nave filled with caring worshipers, asked me if my news were good, bad, or indifferent. I said bad.

He asked for details. I gave him such as I had—the final hospital tests to be made, the surgery to follow. "Who was my oncologist?" It was the first time I had heard the word ("onkos," the Greek word for bulk; "oncologist," the student of tumors). I said I didn't have one so far as I knew, just a surgeon, a gastroenterologist, a cardiologist, and an internist who was also the family doctor. Oncologists, Jim says, are the ones who are supposed to really know about cancer—the cancer specialists. Perhaps I should demand one. The more the merrier.

All this church-going . . . it doesn't seem to have much to do with loving God. Maybe it never did. Fear, perhaps. Suspicion. An effort to placate. Carrying the cross at St. Luke's in Des Moines, the tiny plaster and wood church up the avenue from where Eddie was killed, the church closest to home. Sitting behind Dr. T. on the dais at Central Presbyterian, Grandfather's church downtown; the Barrett brothers, the two who were left, pulpit pages, in identical blue serge suits. Scrubbed faces, slicked down hair. No escape from the dreary interminable sermons, the smug, thin-lipped piety. . . . A decade of questions and indifference, churches for weddings and funerals, nothing else. . . . Then Gerald, the questions answered, the indifference banished. Dozens of churches of every description, up and down the west coast, across the blue Pacific, guttering candles, empty stalls, big, little, high, low, tall, squat, round, square; chapels, cathedrals, meeting houses, temples, anything that might provide shelter for six hours of prayer a day. Five years of churches and then another twenty churchless years until finally, zeroing in, past the zendos, the Trappist monasteries, the upstairs rooms, the meetings of the chosen, the elect, to the cathedral, the little country church, ports in the storm where there was room for everyone.

Still not loving God—defying Him, daring Him to make an appearance, to do His will. A continual provocation, which nevertheless seems necessary for my survival. Although, who knows, it may be love in a different form. An abandonment that is really a closer embrace. The never absent God. The inescapable God. Or as the Sufi parable says: "Your asking God where he is, is His 'Here I am.'"

2. Dr. W., my impromptu psychiatrist—a doctor I hadn't mentioned to Jim—admitted on my fourth visit that widowers were more prone to lymphoma than married men, but little else indicated cancer might be psychogenic. Both he and our family doctor, agreed that surgery was in order and in store, as did Jean S., at lunch, who told me she had had a cancer removed from the gland in her neck seven years ago.

Her story was cautionary. A spiritual malaise had kept her for two years from her dutiful annual visit to a rebbe in Brooklyn. Then something prompted her to go. She met him at 1:00 A.M. (the rebbe apparently sees people through the night). He dismissed her spiritual complaints and told her to get herself to a doctor. The doctor took one look at her neck glands, ignoring any other concern, and sent her off to a hospital, where the malignancy was successfully removed. This all added up, in Jean's view, to some sort of miracle, and in mine as well. The using of His creatures in an atypical way: this is the sort of maneuvering, the imaginative footwork one can expect from God. And there at the end, no more malaise, no more cancer. Back on track.

"If it pains," Jean said, "it isn't cancer. No pain until it is too late."

* * *

NOTHING really stops or changes, although for a few hours over the weekend it seemed it might. Today was a day like any other in the last ten years. My office work—an outline for Oz to use for his remarks in Las Vegas. The *New York Times,* no more nor less dire than on any other day. Viewing Barbara Walters's interview with the Hinckleys—the U.S. TV equivalent of Sophocles, with Barbara acting as some sort of chorus. As my freshman Greek instructor used to say, "Oedipus is just your everyday suburban horror story writ large. It could happen to anyone in Lake Forest or Wellesley Hills."

Then home for a nap and off to Paul W.'s forty-fifth birthday party, where everyone said how thin I looked, which suddenly I am denying emphatically—though a month ago I would have accepted it as a compliment.

3. In his East Side office, the surgeon, Dr. G., patiently explained to me what the situation appeared to be and what I might expect. He was young—maybe early forties—round-faced, dark-haired, pleasant. There was no problem liking him, and he seemed to accept me; at least he laughed at my rather edgy jokes.

I am to check into the hospital on Sunday afternoon. Early Monday I will begin a series of tests to determine whether the stomach is the only area affected. A CAT scan, x-rays, bone marrow tests, etc., etc., and finally—at eight A.M. Friday— surgery. There is no question about that, or that I will lose a half to two-thirds of my stomach. How much else depends on the tests and what they discover when they open me up.

Open me up—the words gave me a slight chill, a sudden sharp picture with me stretched out in its center, a lot of people in white peering in, aghast, amazed. "Sew him back up!" My mother had had a couple of friends who had been sewn back up and left to wait. Better not to have been opened up in the first place. Then the doctor went on making it all sound so reasonable and logical—free of those murky areas where the imagination grows and glows. My cardiologist would be there, standing by, in case of need. Reassuring? Not exactly. The anesthesiologist would take special precautions, a monitoring device inserted in my neck. Why?

Looking back on it, there were enough disagreeable details feathered into his bland, friendly account to convince me he was telling the truth—like the three days of excruciating pain after the operation; the tube stuck into one's nose and reaching all the way to one's stomach, or what was left of it; the dramatic weight loss. Nothing really alarming, but it is better to be forewarned.

Meanwhile a week in the country pursuing the regimen I have followed heretofore—walks, gardening, and other mild exercise; no liquor, no coffee.

Nothing about the ten years off my life that my family doctor has told me at the worst such an operation would cost. If I am allotted the three score and ten, which I have always considered more than generous, that means I am already three years dead.

Water Mill

1. My mind now is fussing with the information I have picked up about my condition, setting it alongside other things that I have heard, to formulate new questions.

What is all this about cancers of the stomach and lymphomas? Stomach cancer, someone has said, is the worst; lymphomas, not so bad. They are talking about removing two-thirds. That seems a lot. They will be checking out other things like liver, spleen, small intestine. As the results come in, if they are favorable, I am presumably expected to find comfort in them, however dire the central fact.

I know from friends, now dead, that hope, no matter how shaky its foundations, is part of the process, and the patient clings to it—if not for himself, then to pass along to those around him who are demanding reassurance. And, of course, there are always the remarkable outcomes of apparently desperate cases—Lou C., Max L. Drastic surgery; heroic measures that worked.

But then I am still secretly waiting for someone to tell me that they've made a mistake. No surgery is necessary.

Or if they do open me up, there will be nothing there; they'll quickly sew me back up, not in horror at what they have found, but in shame at having made such a stupid blunder.

MY prayers are neither worse nor better than usual—cluttered with distractions and near dreams, concerns about trivial things. It is catching up with me . . . just exactly what is involved in all this. I entered this new configuration already profoundly shaken so far as spirit is concerned. I've had a week of support—either from unknown reserves or from a direct tap. I would like to think the latter. But now I am tired. The anxiety is back, and I am feeling a dread of contact that I haven't felt all week, a dread about things that have to be done. Going out to the bank, picking up the papers, refilling my prescriptions, checking about my will, calling the travel agent to cancel Salzburg. Finally, eight years after her death, eight years of dusty waiting in a crematorium in New Jersey, I was scheduled to bring Tilly's ashes home. Now they would have to wait how much longer?

Fussing.

I have six books on suffering in my beach bag.

Alan Paton cites a friend who had both her breasts removed and now has cancer of the spine and yet continually thanks God. I would like to learn from her how she finds the space to insert that thankfulness, me with my paltry little lymphoma of the stomach. Not that you would curse God, but, sensing the origin of the pain, perhaps you could lift yourself somehow above it and toward Him.

> Thou that hast given so much to mee,
> Give one thing more, a gratefull heart . . .
> Not thankefull when it pleaseth mee,
> As if thy blessings had spare days
> But such a heart, whose pulse may bee
> Thy praise.

So wrote George Herbert, who died in his country parsonage in Wiltshire on the first day of March 1633, gently, of a wasting disease, just short of forty, announcing simply "I am now ready to die," asking his wife and niece to leave the room when they wept too audibly, dispatching the manuscript of his poems to his friend Nicholas Ferrar at Little Gidding to publish or burn as he saw fit. Gratitude and trust.

For me, the trick is obviously to accept the fact that my suffering of the spirit (past), of the body (to come) is my own doing. So I get despair, I get cancer, and then, according to the experts, the Reverend Herbert among them, I am supposed to offer it up to God. But God, of course, is the strength that allows me to lift all these self-imposed burdens. It seems inscrutable. It *is* inscrutable. Scrutability, is not, after all, an attribute of the Deity.

According to Paton, Saint Francis kissed the leper and his whole life was changed. Perhaps I am my own leper. What I have tried to do for others, those visits, those little gifts and words of cheer, have been worthless because I have never accepted myself. Or at least, self-acceptance seems to have lagged far behind, and now I may have very little time to catch up.

2. After church I went on to the Southampton hospital to visit sick Episcopalians. Mrs. Halsey, over eighty, suffered a heart attack but apparently is on the mend—a fine woman with a proper society accent, a lot of books of the popular sort around her, and a sense of humor. We talked about the Halseys: the ones she had married into out here on the South Fork plus my two—Edwin and Bull—both characters from my World War II naval past.

Edwin, "the little dancing man" as Gerald referred to him, turned incipient saint, who prayed and played Mozart sonatas and read Saint Thomas and Meister Eckhart in the ward room of his destroyer escort offshore at Tarawa as all hell broke loose around him. A couple of years later he got himself a psychoneurotic discharge—he was caught praying—and came to Trabuco to find God. Too handsome, too bright for anyone's good, Edwin was the one who, speaking out at chores in the kitchen, told the community after a few months coping with the pump, the road, the dying lemons, "You don't use razors to open tin cans." In a day or two, he, the razor, had shaved off his beard, leaving it in the basket in the lower cloister men's room. There I found it, poor lifeless thing, a few days later. Edwin, dead at least a decade, not of cancer or any predictable affliction, but suddenly on some Massachusetts highway in his white Thunderbird with his lover, "unhous'led, disappointed, unanel'd, no reckoning (one suspected, one hoped not) made."

And the other Halsey, Bull, who appeared once in the BOQ in Havannah Harbor where I was a communications officer. He was a tough, mean-looking little man who awed and terrified our senior officers, twice his size, in that Coral Sea backwater. The rest of us didn't register, thank God, on his hard, sharp-eyed vision. What would he have made of a Lieu-

tenant J.G. who didn't eat red meat, drink, smoke, or attend
the movies and who twice, three times a day, depending on
which watch he was standing, took his camp stool, his mimeo-
graphed sheaf of meditations—"God is love, and there are
blessed moments when even to unregenerate human'beings it
is granted to know Him as love"—his pith helmet and mos-
quito net, and set out into the jungle to pray. There was only
relief when Bull, the hero of the South Pacific, took off, in his
flying barge, to some more important outpost. Bull, Mrs. Halsey said—they were all more or less related—came from Elizabeth, N.J., which might explain a lot.

MY second hospital visit was to a tall man in Brooks Brothers
p.j.'s and a silk dressing gown just admitted for possible cancer
of the throat. He was six feet six inches, he told me, and stood
up to prove it. As tall as Aldous, whose cancer was of the
mouth.

3. The afternoon, four hours of it, went in searching for
a picture of Gerald to confirm my memory of his
looks: the beard, the high forehead, the hands. There
had been one of him and Aldous and some others, taken in a
garden in Santa Monica or Beverly Hills. Aldous stooped over
so he would fit in. I never found it.

Instead in a tin trunk full of loose photos and snapshots
were a half dozen of Eddie: Eddie in a wooly snowsuit grin-
ning, toddling toward the camera; Eddie in a beret and shorts
seated with his favorite stuffed animal, a studio portrait, all the
Barrett boys had them taken; Eddie in a kimono and pyjamas,

standing beside the fish pond Dirk and I had dug as a summer project in the backyard on Forestdale Drive, a thoughtful three-year-old, eyes cast down, the last picture, taken the day before he died. Mother had it enlarged and tinted.

There were others of grandfather Will Barrett whom I was supposed to resemble, a tall beak-nosed banker who after grandmother's death always sat in the second row at Greta Garbo films and never gave up his conviction that Shirley Temple was a midget. There was Mary Ellin pregnant with Katherine with the other three grouped around her in the living room in Westport; Mary Ellin with the four of them climbing the rocks and trees in Central Park, the four irrepressible Barrett brats, aged two to nine, and their spectacular mother; Mary Ellin, a wonderful 25, looking sleek and Italian beside the equestrian statue of Marcus Aurelius in the Campidoglio.

The afternoon was over before I put them all back and closed the trunk with a stranger's name painted on the end.

4. Max and Edna came for dinner, having been informed in advance of my condition and prospects. Max, an old cancer hand with an incredibly various and erratic case history, felt an oncologist—that word again—was essential. He swears by his Dr. H. at Mount Sinai, and feels it is Dr. H. who has kept him going—past eighty.

I had never heard Max talk about his cancer and its multiple starts and stops and changed directions, the arrival and departure of symptoms, the uncertainty of the experts. At one time they were set upon removing his spleen, which was so enormous that, although they opened him up, they couldn't get it out. Now, thanks to medication and chemotherapy, his spleen is back to normal size.

Edna feels that cancer comes from some major shock that acts as a sort of organizer bringing together forces that exist in your system, a catalyst. And there are two ways of coping with it. Challenging the disease, like Max, or, just lying back and floating with it, like Lou C.

Then the talk turned to the nature of God. Edna brought up the subject, I guess, or maybe Mary Ellin; certainly not me. Edna quoted Lear—"As flies to wanton boys, are we to the gods; They kill us for their sport"—as representing hers and Max's idea of the deity. She cited the rape of a year-and-a-half-old child as evidence of the indifference of God, as proof that he was "too involved with his grand schemes to attend to such as us." Mary Ellin mentioned Frank G.'s image of an old fellow with a gun sitting on a rocker on his front porch picking off you and your friends as you approach him out of the woods, into the open, one by one. I said rather dimly that I still believed His eye was on the sparrow and that the smallest detail of His creation did not escape Him, which is, for me, certainly as much a terrifying conviction as a reassuring one. But ultimately I feel the reassuring side will win out.

I should have tried to make myself more clear, I suppose, but I have the feeling that such discussions are almost at once off course. God is not graspable or discussable or defendable in those terms. Not that it is bad to natter about God. To consider Him, even in erroneous terms, is better than not considering Him at all. And I would guess agnosticism such as Max's and Edna's and M.E.'s is closer to reality than bigotry or false piety.

I am not certain where that leaves me, who believes but seems to be shut out, barred from any understanding or experience of God, who at best can manage that sort of deep

---

shudder that comes across me sometimes in prayer. And yet I have no doubt of His existence, of my ability, if I truly wish it, to reach Him. That is where the meaning of my sickness and its final cure must lie, in finding and loving God.

BY the end of the evening I had agreed to go to see Dr. H., Max's oncologist, just to make sure that my stomach really had to go. Another opinion couldn't hurt, and then I could make up my own mind. The appointment is set for Friday morning.

5. I got to the beach parking lot a little after six. The sky had a soft band of pink to the east. Mecox Bay was silver and, along its western margin, luminous orchid, yellow, and purple like oily pavement after a rain. And in the eastern sky, high above where the sun was bound to come, was the morning star, the only visible star, bright, terribly bright, so that one could see first a triangle of light, and then the five points with the webbing between, and then what appeared to be a figure with conventional angelic robes, arms outstretched. One could see how the ancients with their active imaginations—seeing whales, swans, hunters, bears, bulls, twins, crabs, where there were only pin pricks of light—might have arrived at angels on high: "Glory to God in the highest, and on earth peace, good will toward men."

In the parking space on the top of the dunes were two cars—a pick-up and a large dingy sedan—and four young men—two, in baseball caps, carrying on an earnest conversation. I waved and started eastward down the beach hoping to see the sun come up.

On the long bar that stretches back from the cut, at the far end along with the gulls was a solitary heron—blue; at least in that light its color was blue. When I was perhaps a hundred feet off, it flapped away. The gulls sat on, craking when the 6:25 train hooted its whistle. The sun came up a moment later, rising from the mist, pink and soft, then fiery red with a dark sash of gray cloud across its middle, then glowing orange. The star vanished.

WHEN I left the beach, the young men were still there, talking. Farming? Girls? Baseball? A friend says, "Cocaine."

MALCOLM, our minister, reported that Mrs. Halsey at the Southampton Hospital had very much enjoyed my visit and, when he told her that I had a heart condition like hers and cancer as well, expressed her admiration that under such circumstances I should still be visiting other sick people. For a moment I felt a glow of self-satisfaction. Then, once again, I realized what had happened. I had been offered my reward here on earth and grabbed it. But I couldn't blame Mrs. Halsey for that.

6. A quote from Norman Cousins's *The Healing Heart,* which someone lent me when my next coronary was still my principal concern: "People who feel locked into objectives that they would rather set aside are candidates for sudden and serious disease."

Here is a partial list of the Cousins's requirements for

getting well: total confidence in my recovery, a strong sense of purpose and even joyfulness, an undiminished will to live, a genuine curiosity about and interest in the treatment, a sense of partnership with the physician.

If this were one of those magazine quizzes that M.E. is forever taking—WILL YOU RECOVER FROM MAJOR SURGERY?—I would score zero.

Still, I have a few things going for me: an undiminished confidence in the continuity of life; a desire to make something communicable out of my present experience, however tricky such communications may be; a stubborn conviction that serving others, even clumsily, half-heartedly, is necessary for my own well-being.

THE New Yorker called while I was out back working in the garden, cultivating the broccoli and brussel sprouts.

M.E. shouted from the kitchen door, and for the length of time it took me to cross the yard, I thought my poem, which I had sent to the poetry editor some weeks back, by some unbelievable fluke had been found acceptable. A whole new career. A reason to survive, as Norman Cousins would have it.

But it was a checker-researcher who wanted me, as an expert on TV documentaries, to tell him something I did not know and who was cross when I couldn't cooperate.

AFTER lunch another visit to the beach. It was windy and bright. A young man with a three-year-old boy stood on the dunes a little way from me. Above them hovered seven gulls, riding the wind, facing the sea. The man was throwing food into the air and the gulls dove for it. The gulls, standing against the wind, hovering in place overhead, were beautiful and mysterious. They didn't flap their wings, and yet they could dart down into the wind and come back precisely where they were before. Finally the man popped what was left of the food into his mouth, brushed his palms together, took the child's hand and walked toward the waves. The gulls wheeled upward and away.

7. Dinner last night with P. and B. Only a few months ago B. was riddled with cancer, given weeks to live if she didn't have additional surgery. She turned her back on her doctors and went to a north woods clinic run by a Frenchman whose methods were so simple and advanced that he had been driven from his native land by the cancer establishment and taken up residence in Canada. His cure amounted to a painless examination of one drop of blood under his supermicroscope. After a three-week course of injections to correct an unbalance revealed by the examination, B. had come home cancer free.

I must do the same, P. and B. insisted. Forget the surgery and all the medical hocus-pocus, chemotherapy, radiation that goes with it. Go north and save my stomach.

Back and forth it went all evening. P. had a nightmare tale of a pal of his who had testicular cancer. Rather than take the time and make the effort to go north, he had had the damn things whacked off, and P. made one of his expressive noises and gestures. B. had a story of a baby with cancer of the eyes. I only half heard it, and couldn't say whether the outcome was happy or tragic. It had to be happy. I don't think one would embark on such a tale—eighteen months old, both eyes—if it weren't.

The whole encounter was like one of those threatening chain letters I have sometimes received which told me the horrible things that had happened to those who broke the chain in the past, and the prodigies performed by those who kept it going. Sickness and death versus hundreds of thousands of unearned dollars, with a vaguely religious cast to deepen the threat, the guilt, if you didn't do what they said. And yet P. and B. had only my own well-being at heart. They wanted me cured, and that made it all the more excruciating.

Finally I said, "Yes, I'll try it." B. said she would arrange the appointment for Saturday morning. I could work it in between Dr. H. on Friday and checking into the hospital, if I still insisted on going to the hospital, on Sunday. A thousand-mile trip. I could leave Friday as soon as I had finished at Mount Sinai.

IT was late when we left P.'s and B.'s, and Mary Ellin and I were both drained and pale. Magic cure or not, the evening had brought me to some sort of confrontation with exactly what I had signed up for next week, which until then I had only half believed. I had contracted to have my stomach removed. I might die. P. and B. knew of many who had done just that—on the operating table and off it after a brief and agonizing period of waiting.

And, of course, there is the problem, which no one brought up, of where the cancer came from in the first place and the heart attack before it, and whether even with a "complete cure," "a clean bill of health," I will have arrived at the real cause and thus prevent another sequence from starting up.

The north woods won't provide an answer to that. Like surgery, it will simply be another postponement.

In addition there is the worry of standing up to authority—going against the people who, if they don't know all about it, pretend to or insist that they do. There is the giving up of the support system that the establishment offers—the approval that I can expect for being a good boy, asking no questions, and doing what I am told. If I go against all that, I shall really be on my own, just me and my cancer—a prospect that scares me out of my wits.

WELL, I have been scared out of my wits before. On my pilgrimage to Laguna Beach to meet Gerald—"the man who knew," who could solve my problems, answer my questions, cure my ills of forty years ago. That was certainly the establishment flouted. An ensign-in-training going four hundred miles beyond the prescribed limit for a weekend pass, on forbidden naval transport. The certainty of a deck court if discovered. The implausible, queer nature of my objective. Who would countenance or understand it. Southern California religion, swamis, lamas, a nest of crackpots. A swimming pool in Beverly Hills, a clutch of starlets, the explanation given my illicit excursion by my navy buddies, a wink and a nudge—that would be forgivable. But I kept right on, down through the terraces of some rich disciple's garden, through his paneled living room, out onto a balcony where Gerald was waiting— Gerald, the clergyman's son, dressed like a bum in a denim jacket, a railroad man's shirt, jeans, and sneakers, with his brindled beard (only derelicts, submarine skippers and George Bernard Shaw wore beards in those days), his eyes like lasers, his hands like calipers, waiting to tell me what was wrong with the world and how it might all be set right. Scaring me out of my wits and then giving me the good news of how to get back into them—the right way round, ready and set for Trabuco. He pointed a thin, flat-nailed finger toward the hills behind us where he was building a house to train us—those of us who really cared—for the millennium, to save the world when the war was finally over—a place to learn how to pray.

There was no comparison, of course, between that grab for salvation in Southern California and this last minute trip to the north. The one was to save my immortal soul, the other to save my stomach . . . and possibly my hair.

STILL, I went home shaken. By agreeing to go to Canada I had become, I feared, not a latter day version of that innocent young ensign searching for the truth, but one of those hopeless, hopeful, live-on-tape people (How many had died since?) whom I had watched on my office monitor heading by the busload over the other border, listening to the double-talk of the people who peddled cure by elixir, cure by coffee enemas, cure by apricot pits, cure by you name it and you could have it—at a price. In Canada there was no specified price for the magical treatment: the final rattling fact. You paid what you felt was deserved, which to my middle-class, middle-western mentality, was the most threatening part of all. What, after all, was my life worth? It was a question that had been asked before.

It *was* Trabuco all over again: far-out religion; far-out science; far-out medicine; far-out anything. We are on the track of truth, the cure; we are the pioneers, the explorers, the ones who really know. If you don't want to buy what we have to offer, to believe, too bad, *tant pis,* fuck you. Go to hell!

There are a million ways to go to hell and only one narrow entrance to paradise. It is your choice. You guess.

THAT grunting opposition to my negative thoughts, which passes as prayer—or doesn't pass—stands there where prayer should be. I am backing into God if I am approaching him at all. It is going west, not south or north, the receding clutter of the track from the observation platform on the old Golden State Limited—a few dusty tumbleweeds, hobos' refuse—and ahead, invisible to me, the glowing bastion of the Rockies pavillioned by marching white clouds and, beyond them, California again.

8. Why can't I handle this malingerer within me as I handle the objects of my charity on Help Line, in the old men's ward in the Jersey City hospital, in the soup kitchen in the South Bronx, in Pennsylvania Station, wherever. I am alert, all attention with the complainers, the ones in desperate need, the people that in recent years I have enlisted to help me act out Jesus' second commandment and those six crucial verses of Matthew 25. If I don't love God with all my heart, my soul, my mind, I can still try to love my neighbor *better* than myself. And I am in no way flattened or defeated by their demands. I am even helpful, cheerful. Why can't I be the same with this clever sniveling wretch who wakes me early morning and accompanies me, protesting, all the way to rising.

So what if I have committed myself to doing something

risky and unorthodox, that the respectable world would not approve? I can change my mind. I can stop fussing.

Fussing, I go to the beach. It has rained and there is no visible source of light in the sky—a layered gray. The sea is coming in in long, cruel slanting waves that blow their tops in combs of spray and rush up the sand in white foam. At the cut there are two surfers in black wet suits with white boards—the first surfers I have seen there all summer. Now that the weather has broken, the sun gone under, there they are, paddling out into those sliding, vicious waves, riding them, lurching, bucking toward the cut, exultant. There is some lesson there that goes beyond the choice between two-thirds of a stomach and a drop of blood.

WAITING for B. to confirm my appointment in Canada, I hacked down the rest of the sunflowers and threw them into the underbrush so that their seeds would not corrupt the garden. I picked the last tomatoes—all green, all fragrant—to ripen in New York, took the last bowlful of raspberries, leaving a dozen more bowls not yet ripe on the canes, and said good-bye to what was left of the basil and the silvery sprouts and broccoli, which are twice as big as they were when I came out a week ago. They seem to be the most successful of all my plants in beauty and strength, and I am leaving them behind unharvested.

B. called. My appointment is confirmed.

Manhattan

1. Max's oncologist, Dr. H., has iron-gray hair. He is wearing a striped shirt and a striped tie. The stripes are bold and go in different directions. He is a friendly, no-nonsense man. From what he has seen of the tests, he is not at all sure I have cancer. Maybe I should have the operation, but the slides don't prove cancer. Let him have a look.

He gives me a thorough examination and sends me back to the waiting room, where an older woman, well dressed, sits with her eyes closed for a long time, expectant, and then without a discernible cue rises and goes out. A young, dark-eyed man—soulful and sick looking—holds a big orange CAT scan envelope. A middle-aged man with gray skin, wearing a white knit cap, and carrying a cane comes in and lies across three chairs. A short stocky man tries to read the paper and gives up, putting his hand over his eyes.

It is different from other waiting rooms. It has a dusty, scruffy underdecorated look—not from neglect, one suspects, but because there are more important concerns, other ways to spend time and money. There is nothing to read. These people around me, I suddenly know, are fighting for their lives.

There is something moist and lumpy and covered with sawdust on the carpet next to the bathroom door.

IN the third hour Dr. H. calls me back to give me his conclusions. Although at least two out of the four people who have studied my slides think I have a malignancy he is not convinced. Dr. H. hatches a piece of yellow scratch paper vertically and horizontally. This is what my stomach should be. This is what it appears to be on the basis of the various interpretations of my slides: nondiagnostic; lymphoma; plasmacytoma; nondiagnostic with a little tail—a "spike." He votes for non-diagnostic without the "spike."

For a moment it looks as though he is going to lift me off the hook.

Still, he continues after a pause, even without a malignancy, even if I think my ulcers are psychosomatic, my own creations, I should have my stomach out. Then they'll know for sure. Cut it out and take a look. Although it may not be too pleasant for me, rather like being hit in the midriff by a Mack truck, Dr. H. says a stomach operation, a gastrectomy will be no threat to my heart and is not nearly so drastic as the by-pass surgery which he had himself not too long ago. He looks very fit.

No malignancy. No stomach. A double negative.

I cancel the trip to Canada, which leaves me with a whole day to kill.

2. There was a baby on a daddy's back at the Morris Graves exhibition at the Whitney, staring over his father's shoulder at the *Instruments for a New Navigation,* the *Spirit Birds.* Earlier, in the park, I had seen another such pair, a daddy with a baby in a bunting, out jogging, big bright blue eyes looking out at me, at everything as they bounced by. Was that good for baby's kidneys, all that bouncing? A quarter of a century ago it wasn't jogging. It was hoisting them all, one by one, on my shoulders, bumping around the backyard in Westport, the rider shrieking with delight, the others shouting, "Me. Me."

There were two more back babies heading into the Met.

The Manet show, for all its panache, was sadder, much sadder than the Graves, for obvious reasons. Graves had to do with eternity—an aperture, small and clear, for you to look through. The Manets were views, singular, compelling, of a life and a time that had long since passed. The note that Manet died of locomotor ataxia did not help to lift the spell, nor did that beautiful final painting of the bar at the Folies-Bergère.

Two kinds of realism. The same reality.

M.E. and I came out of the Manet exhibition into some sort of suburban parade heading down Fifth Avenue: a parochial school band, a float, Miss Cornflower Queen and her court, two young ladies in long white dresses on a flatbed truck from New Jersey, men in short leather pants.

We had a nice New York end-of-summer Saturday lunch, cheerful and light, the kind of lunch we have had since we were two young reporters courting in the same neighborhood thirty-three years ago. I may have changed, but Mary Ellin has very little. She has kept her dark good looks, her Manhattan stylishness, her sharp enthusiasms. She gave me a hard time about Manet. Why should I think him sad? He was the most optimistic of artists. That last painting of the bar at the Folies Bergère done when he was almost dead. Remarkable.

Then we went on to *Fanny and Alexander* which even Mary Ellin couldn't claim as optimistic; which reinforced with a sledgehammer Manet's gentle commentary on mortality or my commentary on mortality stimulated by Manet. Bergman's view of life is skewed, and this time there was more amiss and more left out than usual. But still it sat there on the screen, handsome and hard to ignore, three hours of it. Plenty of things to question, to take exception to. The usual outcry against God and His cruelty. Alexander at his father's funeral saying, "God is a shit"—whatever that is in Swedish. Nothing adds up. A stab at truth and a bewildered drawing back. Not good enough for a final statement, which is what Bergman says it is.

Tomorrow, the hospital. At the eleventh hour I am still asking myself, should I be going?

St. Luke's Hospital

1. I woke at four to an old woman's cries down the corridor, then went back to sleep until the nurse woke me again at 6:30 to take my temperature.

I wonder what governs the woman's shrieks—there are long stretches of silence, and then they come strong and frequent. I am not sure which room she is in. There is an elderly woman across the hall. She looks too frail for such loud cries. A great cluster of colored balloons climbs up her wall.

I had half an hour of prayer, such as it was, after the temperature taking. Prayer subject to interruption. No need for the explanations I dreamed up in the quonset hut, BOQ5 Havannah Harbor. It is obvious that I am lying there wide awake with my eyes closed, not praying, but concentrating on my stomach.

Dr. G., the oncologist—Could he be *my* oncologist?—has now taken a bone-marrow sample, and I have had a twenty-minute talk with him that further reassures me that nothing hasty will be done. He said he would be amazed if I had a plasmacytoma of the stomach. It is virtually unheard of. Lymphoma or myeloma, perhaps. Myeloma. That is a new one.

A visit from the hematologist, then the other Dr. G. drops by. I tell him about Dr. H.—nondiagnostic, not even a spike. Without even a spike, why should I have my stomach out? He tells me if I don't want my stomach out, it won't come out. It will be up to me.

That shuts me up.

THERE is someone down the hall trying to placate the screaming lady. She will not be placated.

DR. W., ravishing in her bright blue coveralls, comes in to tell me that no one seems certain about what is going on in my stomach. I may need another endoscopy.

Miles, my cardiologist, has come and gone. He tells me not to let them cut me if I am not convinced it is absolutely necessary.

MY vanity is fed by the notion that there are so many anomalies in my situation and so many doctors attending to them: "An interesting case." And now the doctors have to admit that they don't know exactly what is wrong. If they discover hard evidence of cancer elsewhere than in my stomach, I tell myself, I will seriously reconsider going to Canada.

A visit from Oz, who has already been to Las Vegas and back. Nothing to it. He tells me that two of his best friends have had their stomachs out and after a few months were eating like hogs and drinking like fish again. Nothing to that either. I don't know whether to feel reassured by the fact that the operation is so common or annoyed at the implication that it hardly warrants all this hullabaloo.

I have been moved. My new room has a view of Morningside Park and the Church of Notre Dame. Out of my window I can see the moon over Harlem and the Bronx. It is orange-yellow and waning. Tomorrow I'll be able to see the sun rise without leaving my bed.

IT is 4:20 A.M. Faraway down the hall I can hear the old lady screaming. It could be tires turned too quickly onto Morningside Drive—almost.

2. Today I am scheduled for a CAT scan of my stomach and adjacent organs at Roosevelt Hospital. Maybe that will tell them exactly what is going on, what alien presence is loitering there. No breakfast. A large glass of orange juice laced with iodine to drink. A release to sign. There is a release for everything. What can happen during a CAT scan? Maybe an accident en route. A collision of wheel chairs. I dress as if I were going to the office.

A bumpy ride downtown. Sitting up in the back end of an ambulance, a pretty paramedic tells me about her single-parent family—her ten-year-old son, a latch key kid. Another subject for a Du Pont Award winner.

* * *

AT Roosevelt, a long wait in a windowless alcove with a photo-mural of New England in the autumn. Then three more tumblers of iodine-laced orange juice and I am led into a low-ceilinged room with a machine in the center and, along one side, a strip of windows with people staring out at me over banks of monitors—mission control or "Good Morning America."

I am laid on a padded slab and they inject me with more iodine. I hold my hands over my head and am slowly devoured. Looking up at the machine, it seems very big—Jonah's whale. Every once in a while it makes a little burp, of protest or satisfaction. I am disgorged. More waiting with New England in the fall.

Finally three teenagers arrive with a stretcher. They insist upon strapping me to it, fully clothed, before wheeling me back to their ambulance. "For insurance reasons." I protest that I have signed a release, that I wasn't on a stretcher coming down. Finally I give in. I haven't the heart for an argument even if I stood a chance of winning. Already at nineteen—a black, a Puerto Rican, a white—they are all fledgling bureaucrats, establishment finks. They wheel me through the corridors, down a ramp and onto the sidewalk. Ninth Avenue above Fifty-eighth Street, midafternoon. A lot of pedestrian traffic splitting to right and left looking down at this strange object: a white-haired man, prone, fully dressed in gray flannels, an olive twill jacket, jodphur boots, wide-eyed, pink-cheeked, with three teenage attendants. Across the way I can see the entrance to Channel 13, where once a year I sit in a dark room with all my downtown buddies putting together my TV program—The Alfred I. Du Pont Columbia University

Awards in Broadcast Journalism. One hundred and twenty minutes of tedium, of glory, depending on where you are sitting. At any moment they may appear—my pals from post-production, from that other racy, nonacademic world: Bob, Gail, Jerry, Judy, Juan, Phil, Charlayne, Isabelle—and look on amazed. "What's going on here? Stand up, man. Stand up." How do you explain being flat on your back in midtown traffic when they don't even know you are sick, or how sick. How sick are you anyway? You don't look sick.

BACK at St. Luke's Dr. W. comes in for a talk. Nothing on the bone marrow, nothing on the CAT scan, nothing to tell us exactly what it is in my stomach except she knows from her endoscope that it is small and on the side.

IRVING brings me a salmon sandwich and some chocolate almond ice cream. He watches me eat it. What have they found out? Nothing. What do they know? Nothing. Come on home.

He gives me a card from his sister: "Greetings from Chartres. The most beautiful church in the world. I hope your ulcer is better. Love, Katherine."

JIM Morton drops by after visiting a young man in intensive care who had been shot through the neck. Some incident in the darkness out there to the east. They think he'll live. Jim reads me three psalms—number 77, number 138, number 103—leaves me his prayer book, and says he'll pick it up later.

In the day of my trouble I sought the Lord;
  my hands were stretched out by night and did not tire
I refused to be comforted.

I think of God, I am restless,
  I ponder, and my spirit faints.

OUT of my window—to the north—there is an unexplained circle of light. Very bright. Black all around. I wait for a long time for something to come into or leave it, some large, hovering, unidentified object.

I go out to the porch to get a clearer view. It is Yankee Stadium still lit long after the game is over.

3. It is 6:15 A.M. From the deserted loggia the morning star is brighter than at Flying Point, and off to the right there is a pale Orion and a pink-rose bank of clouds on the horizon. The bridges have been turned off and the Citicorp Building is glowing white, beginning to catch the sun. Harlem is dark, with smoke rising from its furrows. Two pale cars go down Morningside Drive. The sky is more peach than pink now, with a strip of blue-gray—a wide strip along the horizon for the sun to climb through. A single bird flaps across the sky under the morning star and climbs up until it blots out the star and flies on. Now and then a plane. There is yellow in the sky now and you can hardly make out the red lights on the Citicorp Building. There are three bright clusters of lights directly opposite. La Guardia? There are a few calligraphic clouds above the bands of blue-gray and peach.

The morning star is dimmer.

The big square tower of Mount Sinai beyond the park is the most substantial thing visible—tall, heavy, with few windows lit. The top of Central Park looks narrow and small. A white Fink's Bread truck goes by and a man with a black briefcase disappears under the Scrymser marquee beneath me. A milk wagon. A hospital employee in a green jacket takes the last parking place on this side of Morningside. A police car moves slowly past the entrance. An ambulance heads south. The morning star is pale now, barely visible. The trees in Morningside Park are frailer, less green than the ones farther south. There is gray water visible under the Throgs Neck Bridge and a concentration of brighter sky above where I suppose the sun will appear. At 6:45 it still is not here. A small plane flies across the peach section of the sky into the gray-blue, heading for the three lights.

There is a white line now above the calligraphic clouds which are turning yellow: a pocket of light opens in the bank of blue-gray. The first jogger, in red jersey, heads up Morningside Drive. A bank of pink clouds builds into the blue-gray, but still no sun. Beneath, the color lightens, a V eaten into the bank. The pink is to the north; the blue-gray, to the south. The cables of the Throgs Neck almost meet the pink. The calligraphy above has turned bright, and now you can see an intense red aperture and sense the sun's disk at 6:54, but still not the full arc.

And there it is. First the top with a hint of the lower part through the dark gray streak. Then the full disk above the clouds, shining ochre on a bed of bright orange. The sun is free now with an airplane flying into it.

I can look at it no longer.

* * *

IN *The Asian Journal,* which I am reading, Merton quotes the *Bardo Thödöl:* "Therefore have no fears, have no terror of that deep blue light of dazzling, terrible and awful splendour, since it is the light of the Supreme Way." The date is late and Bangkok and death are only six weeks away.

4. No breakfast again. A stretcher ride instead down long corridors, past the Department of Nephrology, past the Dental Department, into Gastroenterology, where I wait in line watching the doctors and nurses go by. Last night Dr. W. told me that the ulcer itself—there was an ulcer after all—had healed but that the surrounding area still had that lumpiness which had prompted her to take the earlier biopsies. But now, neither the CAT scan nor the bone marrow have confirmed those biopsies. Therefore more are necessary. I lie on my back staring at the ceiling, fantasizing. If this endoscopy proves negative and the upper-GI barium tests scheduled for tomorrow negative as well, I'll make my own proposal: a "natural cure," letting my body and my psyche bring the whole area back to normal. If the doctors miss four out of four, why not give me a chance? I'll simply take off, go someplace for a month or six weeks. Not a resort. Some sort of backwater retreat where there will be absolutely nothing for me to fret about, no one I know or want to meet. Someplace considered too holy for fun and games but not so holy as not to have a few creature comforts—Assisi perhaps. If I could get rid of the ulcer, maybe the bumps will go too.

* * *

AT 9:30 they wheel me in. Dr. W. was waiting to insert the
tube. It took longer than my other two endoscopies. Open,
close. Open, close. The scissors snipped away at the bottom
of the tube. Maybe twenty times. I lost count. Dr. W. said
the stomach looked, if anything, a little worse.

BACK in my room Jim Morton stopped by to give me a
shell, carrot-shaped with bold checks like a gamblers jacket.
I used to find these same shells on the beach in the New
Hebrides—not in such perfect condition.
   Another proof of God's existence, I say to Jim without
embarrassment. As if another, or even one, is needed. Accidental or intentional seems beside the point. If accidental, the
shell, its cunning design, its decoration, then, that, in a way is
even more miraculous, more a proof of God's existence than
if it fitted exactly into some perceivable, carefully thought out
Divine plan. My stomach. The bumps in it. All proofs.

ON Channel 11 I join the Steuben Day Parade, rejoin it
actually, since I recognize it at once as the same parade Mary
Ellin and I walked through last Saturday. There is Miss Cornflower Queen. The St. Ignatius Girls Drum and Bugle Corps.
A group of older gentlemen in blue jackets singing German
folk songs—"I ee, I oh." Clydesdale horses and ten blonde
beauties in braids and dirndls. Another band in blue jackets
and white pants. Bavarian dancers—men holding up ladies,
whirling skirts. A band in orange and maroon uniforms playing "Allahs Holiday"—the final shot.

There they all were and us with them just four days ago—
a beautiful afternoon in New York. Time confounded. Hera-
clitus's stream stepped in twice—thanks to Channel 11.

DOWN the corridor the old lady screams. Her voice sounds
hoarser, more painful. How does she keep it up? It has been
four days since I first heard her.

5. It is pouring rain. My legs ache. I am lying in bed
thinking of Gerald's words of wisdom and warning
that still keep cropping up after forty years, frightening yet giving me grudging encouragement. "You will leave
us here (the little subsistence community of like-minded people at Trabuco), go out into the world, find yourself a job and
a good-looking wife, raise a family. You will forget about the
religious life, and then when you are old and come back to it,
it will be twice, ten times as hard." Gerald the prophet, the
evangelist, the Cambridge Apostle, the man of the world who
knew everyone, everything, had been everywhere, Gerald
calling the shots, scaring you out of your wits and then giving
you the good news and then scaring you out of your wits again.
He knew the month, day, and year World War II would be
over already in 1943; knew all about the atom bomb the year
before that; acid rain, the greenhouse effect; the melting of the
polar ice caps. A real seer—more bad news than good. He sat
there in his canvas chair under the trumpet vine, looking out
across the valley and the green hills and the sea beyond, and
let it all spill out. Nothing rattled him. What he knew. What

God knew. Sooner or later it would all come right. If we wanted it to. That was the trick. To want it.

THE "Hold Breakfast" sign is up on my door again. These mornings when I am not permitted food give a different rhythm to the day. You wake and there is a long stretch with no accustomed interruption, nothing immediate to look forward to. A week ago I could count on prayers, my walk, breakfast, feeding the cat, the *New York Times* to get me started. Here there are just prayers and some new guide in a white jacket and gum shoes to take me to another test. Where is the blood-drawer with his little tray of tubes and his hollow needle and his rubber tourniquet? No blood pressure? No in-bed electrocardiogram? Are they losing interest? Is that a good sign?

FROM the bridge of sighs leading to the x-ray waiting room you can see the cathedral roof, the angel Gabriel blowing his trumpet eastward away from you.

A young woman, small, efficient, tells me not to breathe, not to move. Lots of pictures. With each one the x-ray machine moos like a cow. The CAT scanner—bigger, fancier, more expensive—only made ladylike little burps.

THE tests are finished. Now the waiting. A gray wet day outside the window. The nurse gives me three small yellow pills to clear my system of the barium that, if left unattended, she tells me jokingly, would turn to rock in my intestines.

DR. G. comes in to tell me the barium test is completely clean—no evidence of anything abnormal anywhere. That leaves Dr. W.'s twenty biopsies to go. One out of twenty will be enough to confirm their worst suspicions. Just one. We discuss my options: (1) a gastrectomy on Monday A.M. if the biopsies are positive; (2) exploratory surgery to determine the nature of the stomach's abnormal condition; if there is no malignancy, there will be some sort of surgical procedure to stop the flow of acid into the stomach and enlarge the opening at the bottom and sew me back up; (3) my option—six weeks of right living, right thinking in Assisi, in Salzburg, to see if the bumps begin to go away of their own accord. Dr. G. didn't say no.

AFTER dinner M.E. and I play a game of Scrabble, which we do when circumstances make reading or talking difficult. She wins.

Before we can start a second game Dr. W. comes in to tell me the biopsies are negative, all twenty of them. The Pathology Department is completely mystified at the persistence of the inflamation and the lack of any indication of malignancy since the earlier biopsies three weeks ago. I am to go home tomorrow A.M. Dr. G. will release me. Dr. W. will give me a new medication. I will return for another endoscopy the second week in November. What I do with the six weeks in between is my own business.

* * *

GOD be praised, always. Always. Is that a harsh doctrine? I
think not. I think it may be the origin of real love.
But trusting Him perhaps may be more difficult.

I suddenly realize the lady down the corridor hasn't screamed
since yesterday morning.

II.

In Flight

October

I am on board Flight 844 for Rome. The distance from the head of the aircraft, where I entered, to seat 47-I seemed very long, carrying, as I was, my new typewriter and the heavy bronze plaque that Irving designed for Tilly's grave (Tilly as the nun in Max Reinhardt's *The Miracle*) in addition to all the hand luggage the airline permits me. Tilly's ashes are at my feet in a William Poll shopping bag that held the food for my farewell supper—three salads and some Irish salmon. It is exactly the right size and shape with room to spare for reading material on top: Thomas Merton's *Asian Journals*, Evelyn Underhill's *Mysticism*, *The Tolstoi Reader*, a Helen MacInnes.

WE meandered aimlessly about the field for some time, then, as I read about Merton's religious experience among the giant buddhas of Polonnaruwa, we took off. Now he is at Raffles in Singapore, and everything is black on the far side of the window.

It is odd to read Merton writing in his diary about plans you know he will never accomplish. Indonesia beyond Bangkok: "A whole new journey begins there. And I am still not sure where it will take me. . . ."

Now death is catching up to Merton, in a strangely perfunctory way. No preparation that I can see; no indication that his whole twenty-seven years as a Trappist, his whole fifty-four on earth should be considered a preparation. The writing, the content, the manner is not that of a man ready to leave the world. Plans, always plans. And yet some of his friends and admirers felt his life had peaked there among those massive Buddhist sculptures in Ceylon and that his death—that one brutal stroke, the shock and the shuddering fan falling on him, pinning him to the damp terrazzo floor—however bizarre and arbitrary it seemed, came at an appropriate time.

But something in that view is not quite right. If we must accept our own death, its prospect, its accomplishment, be relaxed about it, we mustn't anyone's else. Nor, though we must be resigned to our own misfortunes, should we find those of our fellows acceptable. I don't know that the book of Job makes that point as clearly as it might, but it is certainly built firmly into the gospels.

Rome

1. At the barrier to meet me, to grab my bags was our daughter Katherine: tall, affectionate, with her edge— not quite of irony—of skepticism about herself, you, the world. The Italians turned to admire her as she led me to the exit, their eyes bulging, unwilling to let her go. Calmly, efficiently she got me from the airport to the middle of Rome. "Diciannove Via Merulana . . . vicino Santa Maria Maggiore," she explained to the cab driver in her laid-back Italian.

THE neighborhood is laid-back too. Not mainstream, not backwater, not fashionable, not dreary, not crowded, not empty, not old, not new, all the buildings of a height—seven or eight stories. The street runs from Santa Maria Maggiore to St. John Lateran. The railroad station is three blocks away. The top of the Colosseum is visible above the buildings across the way. The apartment fits the neighborhood. Big, lots of rooms, tile floors, five balconies, two bathrooms, neo-Biedermeier furnishings, glass doors everywhere, elaborate chandeliers—an upper-level civil servant's family apartment. Three keys to get in: downstairs, the elevator, the front door. Katherine shares the flat with two college classmates. They are out. Katherine has an English lesson to give. I'll read on the sunny front balcony, I tell her, or sightsee in the neighborhood.

I went to the two basilicas, both visible from the front balcony. Inside Santa Maria Maggiore, with its tall, ancient columns, its walls glowing with mosaics, something formidable was in progress: a manifestation of clerics, a semicircle of monks in white, dozens of men in magenta birettas—wave after wave of them coming up behind the altar and kissing it. An aggressive singing of the mass—loud, hard-edged—with the congregation emphatically joining in. Italian Catholicism is difficult for me to penetrate, alien to my northern psyche—bhakti—the path of devotion. Piety you aren't familiar with is hard to assimilate. The religion of the mind, the spirit—not so difficult.

At St. John Lateran an entire village was having its picture taken on the steps, the row of huge stone saints gesticulating wildly from the eaves above the group. Not an entire village, obviously—there were no children—but a large group of adults in their best clothes (rusty black) with a placard (San Marco de something or other) to prove that they had been here and that they had come from there.

2. This morning Katherine and I did the Sistine Chapel and the Raphael Stanze. The Sistine ceiling suddenly seemed quite secular to me. Indeed, the whole Vatican seemed secular. Those endless galleries, the accumulation of works of art and their duplicates and the duplicates of duplicates. How can you tell whether it is the secularization of the sacred or vice versa—the claiming of the world for God, or the corruption of the sacred by the profane? At any rate it seems to have very little to do with the gospels. The hierarchy, the politics, and the art of religion are very apparent—the apparatus, but not the spirit. That doesn't mean the spirit isn't there; just that it is not visible to me. It may be my glands. Where I stand in my own life, thirty years past my first astonished view. Whatever is causing those bumps in my stomach. But I am here to forget about *them.*

3. I am sitting on one of Katherine's balconies getting the Sunday morning sun, looking across a field of roofs, most of them beneath me. To the right an elderly Roman in a bathrobe is hanging out her wash. There is the sharp sound of a hammer against something not wood; there is the smell of burning paper, and directly to the east a man in dark pants and a bright blue shirt and beige sweater is pacing back and forth on what must be a rectory or a monastery roof, saying his office—the first indication of solitary devotion I have spotted in this city where piety comes in job lots. There is something reassuring about this single, thoughtful, slowly pacing figure. On a lower balcony a lady is shaking out her rugs. Bells at a nearby church are ringing. The church bells in Rome don't conform to any clock time that I can determine. Thirteen minutes before; sixteen after the hour.

In the dark courtyard below me four ten-year-olds are playing hide and seek. "Pronto," the boy who is "it" calls out. "Pronto" from somewhere out of sight comes the answer.

Assisi

1. Assisi is rather like Taormina, where M.E. and I chose to spend the first six months of our marriage thirty years ago. Less restless, less raffish, but with the shops, the transients (more pilgrims than tourists, more Italians and Americans than Germans and Danes), even the restaurant bars. But it certainly is not the "Las Vegas of the pious," as one friend who scratched it from his itinerary suggested. So far I am pleased with my choice of a place where lumps might be forgotten or obliterated. The hotel is without bustle or swimming pool. None of those hungry eyes in the lobby seeking you out, trying to place you, or out by the pool in their long chairs observing behind their dark glasses.

Was Mary Ellin right to pass, to say that we couldn't both afford the trip; that after all that had gone on maybe a rest from each other, a substantial rest, would do us both good? However much she loved Italy, would like to recapture our youth, she could wait. I had my experiment to make, a few weeks in peaceful, sanctified surroundings, a complete change. Better to conduct it alone.

I am not sure. Maybe two weeks in Assisi would have put

her back on track. Given her the shove she needs toward starting a new novel. We'll never know.

According to the Rome *Daily American,* I missed by one day a large anti-American rally organized by the Communists here in Assisi to celebrate Saint Francis's birthday. Saint Francis is patron saint to everybody.

OUT of my window I can see two churches and Mount Subasio. Under the window is a table for my typewriter.

2. The drive to Todi, the birthplace of Jacopone, the lawyer turned mystic poet, is by back roads through vineyards and fields of tall plants that could be tobacco—at least they were harvesting leaves, from the ground up, that didn't look edible and binding them into grayish green bales. Outside of Foligno long lines of wagons are parked, heaped with purple and yellow grapes. In the distance I spot Bevagna, Montefalco, and finally Todi, bright on its hill. The day is perfect. Cooler than yesterday, but not too cool, and clear.

I go directly to the main square without a hitch or false turn although I have to thread my way through a maze of narrow streets and alleys to reach it. At one end is the cathedral; at the other, the ancient town hall; cars parked solidly between. I circle and finally find a place. But I can't get the car into reverse to come at it straight; indeed I have been going forward ever since I left Rome. I know where reverse is—to the extreme right and down, hard—but each time I put the gear where it should be, the car moves forward closer and closer to the shiny red Fiat in the next place. We actually touch. Not hard but hard enough to scratch the perfect paint, to make a small dent.

In the glorious, sun-drenched square of Todi (two stars in the Michelin), halfway from the cathedral to the Palazzo del Popolo, with all the male population congregated to take advantage of the sun, the midday break, I have reached an impasse. I can move neither forward nor back. I will never escape. I should never have accepted the foolish, over-sized car; a subcompact would have done very nicely, fitted into the space perfectly. Greed alone had prompted me—something for nothing, more than I paid for. I had only myself to blame. I should never have come to Italy, attempted to escape among strangers, forget my stomach, my heart. I sit there sweating, grunting, trying the gear yet again.

Finally the group of Italian youths who have been watching the whole performance with narrowed, critical eyes—I can see them in my rear view mirror: "What will the stupid American do next?"—come toward me in a pack like something out of *West Side Story*, not exactly snapping their fingers, but with an air of menace, circling. I wait for them to act, to pull me from the front seat, separate me from the ridiculous car that I am obviously incompetent to drive. Now they are examining the car next to me, the bright red one with its new dent. They are bending over it, lifting it, moving it six inches to the right, out of my way, motioning me into the place. I do as I am told.

They move on. Eventually I get out of my car, ignore the cathedral, the municipale, the church where Jacopone is buried, and go off in search of the Ristorante Umbria—one button in the Michelin; "the best in the province" according to *Let's Go Europe.*

* * *

BY the turn-off for Montefalco—"the balcony of Umbria" or, as my local guidebook says, "the railing of Umbria"—I am sufficiently recovered to try again. Another town square, high up, sleepy. A single black sedan with a lady crocheting in the backseat. She tells me to go to the church of San Francesco—every town has one—where, if I hurry, I will be able to see the Benozzo Gozzoli frescoes lit.

An old gentleman in a black suit is showing them to two backpackers with red knees and beards. Saint Francis holding up Arezzo. Saint Francis stripped. Saint Francis zapped with the stigmata, laser style. Saint Francis preaching to the birds. A whole wonderful Gozzoli world, sweet and bright. Umbria as it used to be, possibly never was.

Back at the car a middle-aged man in shirt sleeves summoned from the bar across the square waits to take me up the Torre Comunale. There is no refusing. Everyone who comes to Montefalco goes up the Torre Comunale. We begin the climb, flight after flight, narrower and steeper. What am I doing up here with my faulty heart, my defective stomach, risking my life, what's left of it, keeping up with this fellow half my age who makes his living climbing towers.

And there, finally, at the top, the reason for the climb—spread indeed as beneath a balcony, over a balustrade, all of Umbria, as it is today—Todi, Bevagna, Foligno, Spoleto, Spello, Assisi, and far in the distance, slightly blurred, Perugia.

AT dinner I read the following paragraph from Evelyn Underhill propped in front of me:

And so we get such an astonishing scene when we reflect upon it, as that of the young Francis of Assisi, little more than a boy, asking all night long the one question which so many apparently mature persons have never asked at all: "My God and All, what art Thou and what am I?" And we realize with amazement what a human creature really is—a finite center of consciousness, which is able to apprehend, and long for, Infinity.

And what would young Francis of Assisi, longing for infinity, have thought of me on my querulous pilgrimage through that familiar countryside? What would he have made of me sitting in the corner of my hotel dining room, reading my pious book, while I inadvertently ordered, and then ate, two pathetic, wizened, overcooked little birds?

3. To see the Pinturicchio frescos in the Baglioni chapel in Spello, you insert your hundred-lire note (or your dollar bill) into a slot in a wooden box with a glass top, and as it flutters into a nest of hundred-lire notes at the bottom, the lights come on and there they are: the Annunciation, the Nativity, the Dispute in the Temple, the child Jesus with the eyes of an old man, standing on the tessellated marble of a Renaissance square, sybils looking down from above, the artist himself, observing from a niche to the right, all put there to honor Perugia's first family—yeggs and bullies, murderers and tyrants, every one, who used their own cathedral across the valley for a barracks, who laid waste to the countryside between and turned the peasants into "plundering, murdering savages," like themselves. The evil bribing the talented to evoke the good. In the midst of chaos.

And here am I with my American money bringing it miraculously back. Five minutes and the lights go out.

THEN onto the valley floor where another act of devout obliteration has been performed—Santa Maria degli Angeli squatting like a huge masonry toad over Porziuncola, Francis's cunning little church, where it all more or less began. Two scales: one small, living, authentic; the other big, bombastic, after the fact, diluting, blowing things out of their original properly human proportion.

Not quite. The edifying presence still haunts those hollow, pompous vaults. If we say it big and loud and often enough, how can we forget what once happened here? The carryings on.

SO here I am, headquartered in my cozy hotel room surrounded by all these witnesses, these examples, good and bad, making my pious little tours to the Hermitage, San Damiano, working back in scale to the small, the dark. What am I looking for? Waiting for? Trouble? A cure? Do I really think in the time I have allotted—praying, reading my devotional books, making my pinched little interior comments, sightseeing in this place with its echoes of genuine holiness— do I think I can back out of the dead end I have stumbled into, turn myself around, get this saint with all his documented miracles, His Lord, His God, to haul me out, diminish those lumps that I've never felt nor believed in, actually make them vanish?

4. "In that time and by God's will there died my mother, who was a great hindrance unto me in following the way of God; soon after, my husband died likewise, and also all my children. And because I had commenced to follow the aforesaid Way and had prayed God that He would rid me of them, I had great consolation of their deaths." Thus wrote the blessed Angela of Foligno—a not very attractive town that I have no intention of visiting. "The holiest woman," according to her contemporaries, "in the whole vale of Spoleto."

Our thirty-first wedding anniversary. I talked to M.E. at 11:15 A.M., 6:15 her time. None of my mail has gotten through. Little M.E. is not feeling well. Nothing to worry about, she hopes. A doctor's report today. How am *I* doing? Fine. A nice room. A nice view. Beautiful country. Nothing about the cold sweat I woke into, the three unpleasant dreams I left behind, my depressing reading, blessed Angela and her unfortunate family. "Get rested up. Everyone asks after you. You are missed."

5. Today I took my excursion to Urbino, along the old Roman Via Flaminia. A handsome town—a rich beige; a handsome palace. Somewhere in its bare halls was Piero's Flagellation—the figure of Christ tiny, blurred, but the right, the only tolerable size. Three lounging figures forward on the right, bigger, no one knows who exactly they were supposed to be, standing there, paying no heed. Pilate in the back on the same plane with Christ, staring at him bleakly across an unbridgeable gap, but not really at him, or at the man with the whip. A small world filled with space; timeless—time stopped.

Who is the figure on the pedestal to which Christ is bound? Naked, golden, his right hip cocked, a staff in one hand, an orb in the other. There is no one there to tell me.

6. A Sunday drive through Umbria and Tuscany to Borgo San Sepolcro to look again at what Aldous called "the greatest picture in the world." It has been thirty years since I first saw Piero's Resurrection with M.E. on our wedding trip, sixty since Huxley wrote about it, and its impact has not diminished. There is Christ, the captain of the winning water polo team, and I do mean winning, rising out of the tomb as from an invigorating plunge, flapping his banner above the sleeping figures in the foreground. "They are, you are, you sleepers out there as well," his expression and posture seem to say, "in for a rather nasty surprise." No frozen time, no extra space in this picture ten times the size of the Flagellation in Urbino. A gelid urgency. Huxley, still a fashionable young agnostic when he wrote his description, saw little religion in it. But I, three times his age, have no difficulty in finding in that lowering figure the essential Christ, the triumphant challenger—different from most Renaissance Christs; more like the Christ Pantocrators of Cefalu and Monreale, with their vibrating glare painstakingly built of a thousand shiny bits of stone and glass. Perhaps the eyes are cold, or perhaps they are just looking beyond you, around you, through you at what is holding you back, at what has yet to be done. Not hostile. Not melting. Not really relating to any look I have ever seen on any face that has ever been turned toward me. Unique.

7. There are no beggars in Assisi. I have been here for a week and not seen one. I did see a lot of old ladies looking out of a window in an old-folks home on the way to the basilica, but Assisi seems remarkably free of society's obvious problems. A young punk kid at the band concert last night looking bewildered. Some backpackers, but of the clean-cut sort. No evidence of drugs. Do you suppose Francis's war on poverty, if that was what it was, has succeeded first here. Was that his intention? To embrace poverty and, by embracing it, eliminate it, make it invisible? I rather think not. At any rate, a town whose most famous son's principal love was poverty, has its own hidden away.

PIERO'S resurrected Christ keeps coming back to me. Irving got something of that steady, absolutely honest, truthful, all-seeing, head-on glare in a collage I call the *Tin Angel:* small pieces of pasted paper adding up to that hovering, beetling presence, Hopkins's "Grandeur of God"; and behind the glare, bright wings. It is the face we'll meet one way or another, sooner or later—the unavoidable, excruciatingly beautiful glare of God that means what our lives tell us it means—better sooner than later.

8. To Bevagna for lunch. Another beige town—lower, smaller, poorer. One restaurant open. I consume two more pigeons. This time I know exactly what I am ordering, but I don't want to eat pig. It is not on my diet. Bevagna is where Francis preached to the birds.

* * *

AFTER lunch an excursion into the hills to Sassovivo Abbey. "In a lovely setting overlooking a small valley, the Benedictines in the 11 c. founded their abbey," says the guidebook. "A beautiful Romanesque cloister remains, its semicircular arches supported on slender twin columns. Coloured marbles and mosaics form the decoration. . . . Come out by the Tolentino road. After a half a mile take a little road on the right (sign post) and bear left."

I follow the directions and drive up into the hills. After a mile or two there are a group of parked cars, a path off to the right, a locked shed. *"Euon giorno,"* I say to a young man. He stares back at me, saying nothing. There is a dark grove behind him, no small valley, no cloister. A gun club? Some sort of clandestine meeting? Terrorists? Salvationists? A hunt for white truffles? The residue of the rally in Assisi a week ago Sunday? I drive on. Another young man on a midget motorbike roars round me and up the hill. There is a hiker climbing in the hot sun. Wide views of mountains to the east and west.

Around the bend a large ochre building behind a metal gate. I stop to investigate. A sign on a wall: "The Commune of Jesus." It is locked tight. Blank windows and a sense of being observed from behind them. I back away. The road narrows and climbs between ploughed fields. I drive among muddy farm yards and dirty white stucco buildings up a ridge. The car is too big. I get out and walk until I come to the top, another mountain to the north, a town, no small valley, no eleventh-century abbey. Coming back, below me and the deserted buildings, I see a dozen people—men and women in dark clothes, kerchiefs, heavy shoes—crouched against the earth harvesting a crop I cannot make out.

A wasted afternoon. But in Umbria, on my particular errand, there can be no wasted afternoons.

I saw my first roller skaters in Italy—two boys in the piazza in front of San Rufino. Roller-skating on the cobblestones of Assisi below the ageless pink-gray facade of its duomo is almost as bizarre as roller-skating in the Seventh Avenue subway—the black kid, orange satin hot pants, six foot six if he was an inch, six foot ten in his boot-skates, rolling off the train and swooping, left foot, right foot, great swallowlike swoops, down the tunnel toward Eighth Avenue.

9. Now that they are drawing to an end, what have the two weeks in Assisi meant? A coherent stretch of time set apart from what came before, quite distinct, as I intended it to be. Beyond that, what? The religious element in the environment is separated from my experience, and I haven't been able to make a bridge. Maybe it is because Francis's religion is a young man's religion. I see very few antique Franciscans either in the choir of San Francesco in the morning or in the streets during the day. Middle-aged, but vigorous middle age, and many, many young men in habits. The pilgrims are from a different world too—in large shepherded groups, sometimes American, more frequently not. Even the churches are somehow remote, apart—no matter how beautiful and moving. I do admire San Francesco, am amazed by it, and the facade of San Rufino, but it is difficult to relate them to my spiritual experience.

Here and in Rome, Catholicism still appears a closed,

alien world. I don't belong, and it is important to belong. Nor has there been a religious insight or experience, a therapeutic blast or radiance that might have swept away all those ambiguities that the doctors at St. Luke's and Mount Sinai revealed and then gave up.

However there is a gentleness about the atmosphere here including the religion that has, I believe, served a purpose.

The concierge told me I was *"un uomo tranquillo"*—the calmest guest in the house. I would live to be 150. The last time some one said that was at Trabuco. And shortly thereafter, the rumble and the slide began.

SO if Francis's is not an old man's religion, whose is?

10. Awake at two, in a sweat, my ears ringing, out of a strange dream—a variation on the usual air-raid dream which terminates in a blinding flash. This time the planes flying over saw nothing, dropped nothing. I came out from my shelter and realized that by simply avoiding being seen I had somehow achieved a sort of peace, for others as well as myself. The two warring factions were reconciled. A contested border was resolved. My doing. *Il uomo tranquillo.*

At six I opened the shutters and curtains. There was a clear sky and the morning star over Mount Subasio; and to the west, the moon.

UOMO *tranquillo* or not, there is some sort of desperate struggle going on inside me which could, I suppose, explain the sweating and the ringing ears, if not the dream. I am obviously trying to come to terms with something—a conflict that has been there always and that I've always glossed over, a conflict under a conflict under a conflict. I become frightened and stubborn. I would seem to prefer to die rather than give in, and I am not really certain of what I am fighting for or against. Or if I know, I refuse to admit it. Something has settled in for a last ditch stand and is determined to take everything with it. And something, thank God, seems to be resisting.

I lit a candle in the chapel of Saint Peter of Alcantara at San Francesco for the family, big M.E., little M.E., a good report from her doctor. It is the same chapel where Saint Joseph of Copertino used to take off, praying to the Virgin and suddenly shooting upward through the floor of the main church, through the roof, and off into the blue, out of sight. Then just as miraculously back in place, praying. The Virgin is still there.

Could it be that this abyss over which we seem suspended does not exist, that, whatever our subjective sensations, we are always being borne up, and that Icarus fell in place. No drop, no deadly impact for Phaethon, for any of those noted plummetters, for Lucifer himself. All fleecy clouds above, below. And the levitators—Saint Joseph, Milarepa, Francis himself—the same?

Salzburg

1. All Hallows' Eve. Last night, after three days on the road, Katherine and I arrived in Salzburg. Here we are in the hard-nosed North. Salzburg is every bit as churchy as Assisi, but very this-worldly at the same time. The prince-archbishops obviously were up to their eyeballs in politics and conspicuous consumption. Leopoldskron, the rococo palace where we are burying Tilly's ashes was the summer residence of one of the worldliest.

I have changed from my layered sweaters, gray flannels, and top-of-the-line Nike hiking boots into a suitably sober costume in which to go prospecting in the castle grounds for a proper place to plant Tilly's ashes. They have traveled safely from New York in their William Poll bag—not lost, not crushed, not stolen, not challenged by customs. What would the duty be on the ashes of a former star of stage and screen, a legendary beauty, eight years dead, returning to be buried in her native land? Inside the tightly wrapped bundle was a cannister, perhaps six inches in diameter, ten inches deep, with a top that could be removed—like the top of a tin of China tea. I did not remove it.

MY stomach is making its presence known. Actually I have felt it there for several days. No pain. A thin disklike flatulence that floats up and dissipates itself half way to my craw. I have no notion what that means except probably that when Dr. W. sticks her tube down my throat in a week or so the situation will not be improved.

November

2. I wake in the dark in my small, folksy-elegant chambers at the Goldener Hirsch. It is All Saints morning. My bed is damp, with fear, not love. I am back to that July afternoon fifty-five years ago. That granted prayer. "Go fetch your brother, Marvin." "Why? I'm busy. Why do I always have to do it? Why can't Dirk? You are interrupting our game." "Go on." "I don't like Eddie. I wish he were . . ." The last inaudible except to me. Eddie dead. Eddie the prettiest one, the most cheerful and willing. The brightest. Who could resist him with his dark curls, his dimples, his ready smile. Out of the way. The favor transferred back to me, the next to the youngest. Never.

Where did that Essex sedan come from? Tall. Gray. Deadly. How can I ever see its impact as an act of love and not as one of punishment—instant retribution—sending me screaming and whimpering down the hill, down the years, compensating, punishing myself, others. One feels the thinness of the separation. Salvation there. Me here. Thin and constant. One choice, one honest act of will, of contrition would penetrate it like a fist through paper. I've known this, or maybe just guessed it, for years, for over forty years certainly, and yet, I cannot make the fist, let alone raise it, strike. The thinness, I tell myself, is me, me standing in my own way. To confess that awful error, that deadly wish, to admit and then repent it would be to invite my own death. Marvin, dead, not Eddie. And so I go on sweating, struggling.

I turn on the light, and across the peach-colored room—blush-yellow, the inside of a peach—beyond the foot of the bed, under a lampshade bright with delphiniums, tulips, anemones, sits Tilly in her can.

AT 8:25, when the bells began to ring, I was in the University Church. I walked out of it, past the Franciscan Church (closed for repairs), toward the cathedral, into the heart of the bells—bells all around me. What a glory! And why not? Who better to celebrate with bells than all the saints. Those we have heard of, and those we haven't.

TOMORROW we bury Tilly.

3. All Souls Day. Before breakfast I pried open Tilly's ashes with a combination of my nail clippers, which broke, and the Goldener Hirsch room key. The tin was not quite full. Two layers of crepey beige paper on top. The ashes were whitish and more in flakes, less dusty, than I expected them to be. I left the top loose in case it was decided that I should scatter them rather than bury them.

TILLY, the glamorous, the naughty, the talented, Tilly, our family friend is finally buried. It was a beautiful day. The priest, a plump, jovial man, not young nor old, appeared a little before ten, and we all gathered out by the pedestal beyond the castle terrace where the gardener had dug a hole. Katherine carried the roses and I the plaque and ashes. Benjy, Katherine's boyfriend, who just arrived from Spain, took pictures for those other old friends of Tilly's who weren't able to be present. At the appropriate moment I knelt and deposited the ashes in their tin at the bottom of the hole. The priest blessed them with a green twig and holy water and the gardener covered them with earth. The service—in German, with me saying the Lord's Prayer in English—lasted perhaps ten minutes. For a moment I couldn't remember the words that were as much a part of me as my teeth, that I'd had almost as long. Then they came back to me.

Out to the left were the stone horses, the landing where Julie Andrews and all the Trapp kids had tumbled out of the boat to meet the cool gaze of Christopher Plummer and Eleanor Parker dressed to the nines. The lake is empty—a wide expanse of gray, fetid mud.

4. A dream that ended with me on roller skates speeding downhill. Roller skates again. In front of me were logs, big, substantial logs. I flipped them out of my way with something thin, flexible in my hand as I sped on. A cane? An umbrella? It was all managed with incredible dexterity. The flipping—the light wand dispatching the heavy logs, scarcely bending. There were pedestrians. I missed them, one after another, barely, swooping around them at high speed. An old woman crossed my path and was gone. Nothing stood in the way of my exhilarating triumphant progress, a clear run ahead of me. And then I woke. This morning I leave Salzburg alone.

Katherine and Benjy have returned to Rome.

Paris

1. Linda, Mary Ellin's middle sister, small, straight, was waiting yesterday at the baggage claim at the airport. I spotted her there a block away. I think I could see Linda through a brick wall. She has that kind of intense, focused beauty. She barged through the barrier the moment she saw me, ignoring the protests of the customs officers. For a supposedly timid woman she has admirable spirit. Nothing for the customs men to do but shrug their shoulders.

I woke before the household and let the prayers go on for an hour. I seemed to be getting somewhere, somewhere both frightening and reassuring. It was like going up steps, one riser at a time, bringing the second foot up to the level of the first before stepping on—the stair climbing of the very young, or the very old, with no idea, no conception of what is waiting for you at the top.

2. Chartres. The weather good but not perfect; overcast at the end. The church standing there far away across the open fields, coming closer. It alone, still, the horizon's only interruption. Heartbreaking, the sight of it, taller and more solitary, it would seem, than any building in Christendom.

I am aboard a monstrous 747 with its gnu bump at the shoulders. Takeoff is at 1:05. There go Paris, Salzburg, Assisi, Rome, and all the rest into a dirty mist.

III.

New York

1. This morning M.E. told me, somewhat uneasily, that Dr. Southworth, our family doctor, wanted me to call him immediately. He had not been happy about my getaway to Europe. "If I had had those ambiguous slides," he said to M.E. a few days after I departed, "I would have gone through with the operation. You can have fifty negatives and one positive, and it is that positive that has to be attended to."

When Dr. Southworth came on the phone, he said he wanted the results of the next endoscopy immediately. He repeated what he had said to M.E., adding that I should have the operation whatever the new endoscopy says.

So we begin again.

A daydream—half asleep, half awake. I am invited to occupy the pulpit at St. John's. In procession behind the incense, the shining Bible, and the Cross, I am led up to the steps and mount alone, walking slowly in my university gown. My big chance to tell all, to give the word, the example. I look out at a cathedral full of lifted faces, quiet, expectant. All I can do is weep—no words, just tears.

* * *

ANOTHER daydream. I have refused surgery. I have told them all—plenty of words now—that, if indeed it is cancer, I am convinced that it is me who is the cause, and there is nothing they can do. Nothing short of setting myself straight will satisfactorily dispose of the malignancy either in a cure or death. To submit myself to a series of processes aimed at improving or eliminating the condition mechanically, arbitrarily, no matter how cunning or resourceful, would be a waste of their ingenuity and what time remains to me. I am emphatic.

After lunch I call Dr. W. and set up my endoscopy for Wednesday at one.

2. Elizabeth's birth day—thirty years ago. Our first child. Mary Ellin dopey in a room full of flowers. Then the nurse held the tiny thing up to the glass and reality took over. Three of us. The family had begun.

Elizabeth sounded fine on the phone. Thirty obviously didn't faze her. Why should it?

"How are you, Daddy."

"I'm just fine."

"How was the trip?"

"Terrific, incredible." Those adjectives again.

THE view down my esophagus, said Dr. W., in that dry drawl of hers, was much worse. She tried to give me a look at my stomach, but I saw nothing when she handed me the top of the tube—a blurred stretch of nothing, maybe gray, maybe reddish, maybe smooth, maybe bumpy. Impossible to tell; nothing to compare it to. I'd never looked at the inside of my stomach before, or anyone's else. I don't care to again. But in a few days maybe, if they, the medicine men and women, have their way, there won't be anything to look at.

As for those twenty biopsies that launched me on my trip to Assisi. They weren't, she tells me now, as negative as I had assumed; ambiguous at best. So it seems we are back, if not where we started, at a spot farther along, heading in the same direction.

At the earliest, Dr. W. said, the operation would be scheduled after Thanksgiving.

BY going to Assisi I gave God space, I thought, a chance to work a miracle—the angry red gone, the bumps smoothed out. He didn't choose to take it. So I am committed to the other path. What would you call it? The nonmiraculous, the nonmagical. But do I have it quite right? The miracle is there on the stretcher, on the table under the lights as well. Flat on my back, down on my knees—only the instruments change. The end is the same.

As for Canada—the real hocus-pocus, man putting one over on God and the doctors alike—that I don't even consider.

A zen question via Thomas Merton: "Where do you go from the top of a thirty-foot pole?"

My answer: On to the top of the next thirty-foot pole. And the next. And the next. No fall. No ascent. A forest of thirty-foot poles . . . until, suddenly, there are none.

Water Mill

1. One five-subject notebook filled. Another begun. Half legible even to me—the Palmer Method corrupted by time, never thoroughly grasped, although I would have done anything to please Florence Sullivan, my red-headed fifth-grade penmanship teacher.

Now my scribbling gets first place every morning, before my prayers. From necessity, not choice. Otherwise the prayers would be a tangle of recollections, "profound" thoughts, observations. For all I know, I am gathering a harvest of weeds for someone else to sort out. One of those logs kept by the captains of derelict ships, doomed wanderers in the desert, mountain climbers lost above the timberline, men in lifeboats, men huddled, writing beside wrecks of one sort or another in some kind of wilderness. Maybe it is just a catalogue of mistakes that others can avoid. An account of futile persistence—bravery without issue—or cowardice without cause. The meaning depends on what happens next . . . last.

Things have obviously changed since that year back home in Iowa when I was in flight from Trabuco, when I couldn't bear to think of God, of the world, of either one; when soap operas and stories in *The Saturday Evening Post* were the closest I dared to approach reality, the farthest escape. All I was able to write then was a check to cover my bank balance in my parents' favor in case I should be found senseless—mad—in my attic room. A few hundred dollars that might help to dig me out. Still hope. A year of desperate hope.

LAST evening I looked up the essay on Pascal in the encyclopedia to find out how old he was when he died—thirty-nine—and remind myself of that sudden blazing of the spirit which he recorded in a brief memorial "From half-past ten till half-past twelve, Fire!" But instead of a description of that dazzling, life-changing experience, I found myself reading about his dying in agonizing pain of cancer of the stomach. Was that the fire? Not at the apex of his spirit, but a prophetic gnawing at his gut. But I tell myself what I have is something quite different, not cancer *of* the stomach, but alongside it, around it. Lymphoma caught soon enough is quite curable—by surgery, by radiation. That is what they tell me, but I don't listen. I don't believe what they are saying. It is what they told T., and C., and B. and B.—what they tell everybody, true or not. The only thing to believe is your gut, and right now mine is sending the wrong signals.

WHEN I came through the living room this morning on my way to prayers, there was a log still glowing in the grate—fire!

2. A party at the P.s'. Timothy drives us over in his big green coupe de ville. The usual words of cheer. The embrace. A lot of people talking shop—writing shop, painting shop, real estate—but I occupy the whole horizon. A great lump blotting out all else in my twill jacket, flannels, and the linen shirt M.E. and I bought in Innsbruck thirty years ago, a heap to be climbed over to get to the others, and I don't have the assistance of drink to boost me over. I am still honoring the ulcer.

I find myself in a discussion of the miseries of old age— friends of the host's, the man stashed away in a nursing home, miserable and alone, his wife miserable and alone in their big village house. The pain at the end of life seems almost as hard to explain as the mortal afflictions of children. The answer, of course, is constant, exactly the same. In between as well. But who will even bother to put the question . . . and then listen.

3. M.E., who had business in town—getting a new free-lance editing assignment and turning in an article on abused children—came out on the 7:02 train. We had dinner at the Mexican restaurant next to the Southampton station—a noisy place with a dart board, a juke box, a TV set, electronic games, all in simultaneous use; all the tables, the bar filled. We sat next to two young men in their mid-twenties. Hearty, red-faced jocks in plaid shirts. Except, when I looked again, one young man had no hands, only two metal extensions which he used to eat and drink; the other was blind.

No one paid them particular heed—not the waitress, not the other patrons. All the noise and confusion insulated them, rendered them invisible, sparing them comment or concern. Maybe that was why they were here. Maybe that is why we are all here in this noisy, cluttered, busy middle world—so that our handicaps won't show.

We had combinations. One tostada, one tortilla, one enchilada each. So much for my stomach.

4. Thanksgiving at Alton and Elizabeth's—a pretty old house deep in Connecticut, a hillside of dark evergreens, a red barn, fires in the parlor and library and dining room. The perfect setting for the holiday, almost too perfect, too much to be thankful for. Family. Friends. Elizabeth Peters, M.E.'s youngest sister, tall, elegant, has repose and a considerate husband. It is an unbeatable combination when you are having fifteen for dinner and no kitchen help. Besides, she is a wonderful cook.

Turkey; dressing; puréed chestnuts, creamed onions, cranberry sauce, scalloped potatoes, leeks, zucchini, and carrots; pumpkin, mince, and apple pie; plum pudding; nuts, mints, a chocolate turkey at each place. I ate everything. My last Thanksgiving with my stomach intact.

What will Thanksgiving without a stomach be like? I wouldn't ask myself that question if I didn't think I'd have an opportunity to answer it.

* * *

"IDIOTS and lunatics are remarkably exempt from cancer in every shape," a nineteenth-century doctor observes in the book I am reading. "Distress of mind," not lunacy—he makes a distinction—is the first cause. "Exhausting toil and privation" come next. So the rich meet the poor in suffering and pathology.

New York

1. Mary Ellin's birthday treat: Peter Brook's *Reader's Digest* version of *Carmen*. No treat. I kept trying to extract some universal message—Brook always has a universal message—but it wouldn't come. A lot of abracadabra without any magic. Gritty, dry, with an ending even grimmer than the conventional one and less convincing. Instead of a doomed spitfire fighting and defying her rejected lover, she lets him lead her, unprotesting, to her death. That is the way it was in the novel, we are told; the opera was a melodramatic lie. I prefer the opera.

THE Right Stuff with Irving. A great big handsome movie. More raw material here for working over than in Brook's *Carmen*. The reminder that there is a stretch on the way to outer space, on the way back, where you are no longer in touch, where communication is not possible.

December

2. A brand new hospital, Columbia Presbyterian. A brand new doctor, Dr. H., the best in the field, I am told. Not so new, it turns out; he was in my class at Harvard, on the crew. Tall, pleasant, obviously intelligent, healthy. I told him my story. He took notes, gave me a brief exam, and said he would call me tomorrow A.M. with his recommendations. "There is," he said, "no cause for anxiety." Perhaps, if "there is no cause for anxiety," I should forget about the operation.

How often can you be told you have cancer and still get this uptight waiting to be told yet again? When will you finally believe it?

I am killing time, reading *Vogue,* which is mostly ads. Page after page of expensive trash. At the back of the book a bright spread or two. A wicked waste of talent, of paper; every page should be bright, I tell myself crossly. No waste. No boredom. For someone with proper vision, the Christmas issue of *Vogue* should be a book of hours, the Oxherding Pictures, the windows at Chartres—revelation after revelation. I let the magazine drop onto the quilt and stare out our bedroom window at the dirty bricks opposite.

MARY Ellin asked me to please have the operation any day but December 13, the day of M. and A.'s thirtieth wedding anniversary party. One day before, one day after would be fine. She wants to wear her beautiful new dress. It was intended as a joke to cheer me up. I didn't find it as funny as I should have. And beneath her joke, her pretense at frivolity,

there is another reason. Her husband, her best friend, both
with cancer. If she didn't laugh, she'd weep.

3. Sometime during the night I admitted to myself that
I might never make it. And that doesn't mean survive
the operation. That possibility doesn't seem particularly to interest me. Making it, so far as I am concerned, means
growing up—coming to terms with reality—and then, once
I've done that, adjusting myself to its needs, serving it. When-
ever I feel I am getting near that state, something seems to
intervene. And now I am using this illness in some peculiar
way, perhaps to test growing up, but more likely as a last-ditch
effort to escape the necessary confrontation, to put it off yet
again.

I have built my life in the lee of the blast, protected from
reality, not facing it. That conversion, which would bring me
out into the real weather, has never taken place, and what I
have passed off as religion is simply a variation of self-protec-
tive worldliness. At Trabuco I peered around the corner,
caught reality's edge, and my whole concern became to get
away as quickly as possible—to distance myself from that roaring blackness that I had been told was really light.

And so now all these years later I am peering around the
corner again, with no prospect of a second escape. Will I go
through the blackness and come out the other side? Will I
make it?

THE date for the operation is set: the morning of December 12. The next evening M.E. can go to M.'s anniversary

party and wear her new dress and give them all the good news. No good news, no go. We don't even discuss it, think it.

DR. W. now says the smears are *very* abnormal and definitely, unequivocally indicate a malignancy—something about lambda cells and proteins I couldn't follow, didn't particularly want to follow. Lambda, plasmacytoma, lymphoma, myeloma—all names for sports cars that old-time movie stars used to drive.

SO now the question is not, "Is it cancer?" but, "Exactly where and how much?"

I walked over to the cathedral, up the steps and down the nave, around the apse, and out again. Then over to the office to tell Janet, my second in command, and Oz. Janet told me about her husband Larry's two twelve-hour operations, every lymph gland in his body, it sounded like, removed, and he was back playing baseball in the park a week after the second. Oz said, "Let's wait and see."

I remember one of M.E.'s mother's favorite observations. "In your twenties you call your friends up joyously and say, 'It's a boy.' After fifty you call your friends up joyously and say, 'It's not cancer.' "

Not always.

4. Dr. E., recommended by the Jung Institute, is eighty-two and lives in an old-fashioned apartment on Central Park West. I was there to see if he could guess exactly what I am doing to myself and if a follower of Jung could think of a better, more creative, less lethal way for me to do it. Freud had had his chance—several times.

The interview lasted a full hour; no nonsense about fifty minutes. His advice was to put the energy I am now misusing in apprehension and gloom into healing.

Maybe he helped. At any rate, I was able to walk the fifty-eight blocks home.

He doesn't bill, but has you put your check in a little homemade box with a slit on a table in the waiting room—just drop it in, like in the lira box in the Baglioni chapel in Spello but without the illumination.

5. As a consolation prize for missing her party, M. is taking me to the opera: the Saturday matinee of *Dialogues of the Carmelites*. Second row, center. At the end of the first act, there it is, the ultimate horror set to music. The woman of God, the mother superior, dying a bad death, the worst. A failure of nerve, of faith, the fear of the pain, the fear of what comes after, the ultimate humiliation with all those little nuns, her daughters-in-god, as witness. It was her stomach. Cancer of the stomach. Writhing on her hard narrow bed. "God has become a shadow."

IN the entr'acte in the Grand Tier restaurant, M. ate shrimp wriggle with black bread and butter and a crème caramel, and

I had two cups of tea, no cream, no sugar—nothing but clear liquids, Dr. H.'s assistant had told me, between the opera and the operation. The two of us, both with our own cancers, discussed other people's deaths, her mother-in-law's, her father's, again both of cancer. She had witnessed her father's, and marvelled at her own mother's spontaneous response to the death of her husband of more than fifty years: crying out a prayer, thanking God for what he had given her, her husband, her children—a single affirmation that had to be at the same time a protest, a shout of pain binding all those years together.

Back to Act Two. More deaths. Young, clean-cut, the little nuns refusing to renounce their vocations and declare God dead, reaffirming His existence by marching calmly to the guillotine, one by one. The *Salve Regina* finally silenced, voice by voice. Death by choice.

AT the Pierre we looked into the ballroom, where they were already preparing for the party on Tuesday. Flats along the walls representing M.'s boat, the Greek Isles. Bright colors. Bustle. It looked like it might be fun. By Tuesday I would know the truth about my stomach.

6. I woke some time after 1:30 with the horrors—a black wall that I couldn't penetrate or clamber over, a black wall that swayed. There followed hours dominated by darkness and dizziness. Somewhere, I told myself, in all the clawings and scrabblings, half-aspirations, weak intercessions, scuttlings along the bottom trying to find a way through, was a half hour of prayer.

Finally at nine I bumbled out to feed the cat—swaying and lurching—to have a glass of cranberry juice (permitted), some tea, vitamin C (no one said anything about vitamin C on the morning before the operation), and to retrieve the Sunday paper from the back landing. Then shaved, took a bath, read the paper. In the mirror I looked eighty—gray-faced; hollow-eyed.

The phone call came from the hospital at 10:40 suggesting I appear at 1:00.

There was no question of church, of the communion Dr. H.'s assistant gave me permission to take when I was impertinent enough to ask, "What about the wafer and the wine?" It would have been a heroic thing to do: staggering across College Walk, down Amsterdam; creeping up the steps, down the center aisle all the way to my usual place in the fourth row; singing the hymns; lining up. But who is a hero?

WHILE I was reading the paper in the living room, the cat, which had been skulking in the back of the apartment, suddenly shot out of the pantry door, raced the full length of the dining room, picking up speed, leapt across the sofa where I was sitting and landed on the jade tree, splendid and glossy green, which was on the window ledge behind me, then made a second wild circuit of the room, hitting the plant once more. This time the cherished plant (given to me by my mother-in-law to celebrate my return home from my heart attack four and a half years before) went over onto the floor, and the cat ended up behind the sofa in hiding.

The ruined plant has now been put out with the trash on

the landing, and the culprit and I back in the bedroom are both sitting at the end of the bed viewing ourselves in the mirror with no visible trace of wickedness or mischief about us. My color is back and I am sixty-three again.

In another hour M.E. and I shall set out for the hospital.

A question for tomorrow morning. What will happen when my spiritual wallowing meets up with real physical pain? Not that the wallowing isn't real in its way and painful. But I have the illusion that it is something that I can do something about. Perhaps I can do something about the pain too.

Columbia Presbyterian

1. M.E. arrived at nine. She held my hand and asked if I were frightened. "No. Not at all," I said.
I'm not.

2. No pain killers for two days. Last night no sedative. There is a stapled incision down my stomach—ten inches bisecting my navel, with a few more stitches above than below. No sense of intrusion or loss. I can sit to pray.

The world outside my hospital room has an unreal hallucinatory quality reported on by M.E. in her long daily visits: M.'s gala, a great success; Lily's first birthday party, bigger than M.'s gala; a dinner at the A.s'.

It is almost as though I got sick on purpose to avoid it all: the food and drink, the talk, the toasts, the confusion. But it is unavoidable, the world. There it is on TV. Malcolm Forbes and Louis Rukeyser in a special Christmas edition of "Wall Street Week" celebrating all of Malcolm's possessions: his toy boats, his Fabergé eggs, his motor cycles and yachts, his French chateaux, his balloons. Allusions to the magi, frankincense, and myrrh. Gold. Mostly gold—the necessary ingredient. In questionable taste, but what isn't at this time of year?

There have been a lot of flowers. A lot of phone calls: my children, a nephew and niece, my brother, my brother-in-law, Mr. B. "You need to take care of yourself, Marvin," said my father-in-law. He is entitled. He has made it to ninety-five.

AFTER lunch Elizabeth and Sasha, just in from California for the holidays, arrived along with my nephew Dirk, who was carrying a shopping bag with a plate of homemade cookies and a pink poinsettia. The young men, from my prone position, looked particularly fit and handsome. Elizabeth, wearing the amethyst and crystal beads her mother gave her for her 30th birthday and a sweater the color of Concord grapes, has an elegance about her that belongs neither to the East Coast where she was born and raised nor the West Coast where she has lived for the last decade. It is all her own which I guess could be said about any true beauty. Unique. All my daughters are beauties—like their mother, like their aunts, like their grandmothers, like their great aunts, like their great grandmothers. Why is it that every woman close to me turns out to be a beauty, or is one already. Should I take the credit?

Morningside Heights

1. I am out and in the clear, sort of—me and all the poinsettias (four), cyclamens (two), African violets (three); the cut flowers are left behind—out through the lobby, tiles below, a coffered ceiling above, out the revolving doors under the porte cochere (a trip I have made before with M.E., four times, four different babies, not that different, all wrapped up with only their wizened pink faces showing). Into the backseat of the dark blue Chevrolet with Sasha at the wheel, ten minutes down the West Side, and home, minus the distal half of my stomach, my pylorus, and half an inch of duodenum as well as a few lymph glands in the vicinity. My prognosis: "good." Not "excellent," not "very good," but "good," like in the Mimi Sheraton restaurant ratings. One star, not three. Better than "fair." Better than "unsatisfactory."

In the bathroom mirror I resemble the soldier who had been caught in the Utah atom tests as he appeared halfway through the TV mini series—down eleven pounds, and it shows.

I have that gray, washed-out, luminous look in the bedroom mirror as well—the look that I have always interpreted as the I-know-I-am-dying-and-I-don't-like-it look, except that it is nothing of the sort. I have known that death was imminent and inevitable since childhood, and I have risen pink-cheeked, round-faced, bright-eyed above that knowledge like a kite above a gusty wind, rising and then diving into it, barely clearing the ground before I rose again. This look I have now is the I-have-just-suffered-a-grave-insult-to-my-gut look, or the six-goddamned-hours-under-the-anaesthetic look, or the ten-fucking-days-without-a-decent-meal look. It has nothing to do with death—or no more than any look I give or gesture I make.

2. It has been ten days since the operation, and now it would seem I am someone who has had cancer just as I became someone who had had a heart attack four and a half years ago. I am sitting, waiting to hear how much of a cancer and the prognosis—the real one "based on the pathology"—but otherwise the whole experience is drifting into the distance like something dropped from the fantail of the ship that took me to the South Pacific, twelve days out of San Diego. No Jap submarines, no alien aircraft. A lot of flying fish, a porpoise, an albatross or two. Me and two or three thousand others below decks. All through the war, those flirtations with death, like some adolescent waiting outside of Sardi's, to catch a star's, any star's, eye—not a chance. I waited for the Aleutians in Seattle, and they sent me to the New Hebrides. I waited for the Solomons in the New Hebrides, and they sent me to Hawaii. I waited for the Ryukyus in Hawaii, and they sent me home. At home I waited for the chain reaction that would consume us all, and it stopped on

Honshū and I was free to spend my life as I saw fit—or so it seemed.

BROTHER Dirk, handsome and prosperous, here from North Carolina to be with his children and grandchildren for the holidays, came to see me. He kissed me good-bye. In a family where men do not kiss, what did that mean? The kiss of peace? There had always been peace between us. The kiss of farewell? Did I look that bad? A feeling of sudden tenderness, perhaps, for that little brother to whom he had always been a protector and friend and who now might die out of his proper order. I didn't ask for a reason, but gave him a hug and let him go.

3. Christmas Day. Sometime during the night the smoke alarm's failing battery began its cheerful terminal chirp; the little black cat in heat prowled the hall, wailing.

A dream. An outdoor party, not on a lawn—in an open space with a tall fence, a ditch, a railroad right of way. People at the party surprised to see me. Me aware for the first time that I can recall in a dream that I am dying—not threatened with death, actually dying—different from all the dreams in which I am about to be overwhelmed by catastrophe—atom bombs, tidal waves, hurricanes—and yet survive. In this I am mortally ill . . . and alone. The other people at the party are over there, and I am sitting on a sort of stile, eating an apple, wondering how to dispose of the core.

At six I get up to feed the cat. I find her sitting on the

dining room table alongside—exactly parallel to—the Christmas turkey which was set out last night to thaw. I put the turkey into the oven (unlit), fill the cat's water bowl, and open an envelope of Tender Vittles, then go back to the bedroom to pray.

All the family—M.E., Elizabeth and Sasha, little M.E., Irving—everyone except Katherine, who is still in Rome, was here for breakfast. Little M.E., looking pale but on the mend, in good spirits. She could make the seventh of the Kruidenier children, my mother's family—six young faces, each in their allotted oval in the old daguerrotype, the same finely drawn visionary good looks. Not the sort you necessarily associate with the Dutch, but Dutch nonetheless.

We opened the presents. For me, a heather blue sweater with raglan sleeves which Elizabeth has been working on for three years, ripping it out, starting over again; the quartets of Beethoven, all of them; clothes; books; ties. It seemed to me I had more and nicer presents than anyone else, than I'd ever had before in my life.

4. Dr. H. called to report the latest on my stomach, or what used to be my stomach. They now feel it was (is) not plasmacytoma but strictly lymphoma (no mention of myeloma) and that, of the additional biopsies taken during the operation, four lymph nodes give evidence of malignancy. I have no idea how big a lymph node may be or how many of mine were extracted to find the four naughty ones. He didn't tell me and I didn't ask. His recommendation is a course of radiation therapy—three weeks of daily visits, which should begin as soon as possible. That resolves one question—Exactly what was in my stomach?—but leaves me uncertain about the "goodness" of my prognosis. One star, and possibly, since one lymph node has been upped to four and radiation is recommended, we may be verging on no-star territory. Fair or worse.

Meantime, what about my heart? How is it holding up and how will it hold up? I am reminded that I am hanging on two hooks. The heart attack hook, four years in the wall, and the cancer hook, just screwed in.

A message on the new answering machine, one of our Christmas presents. Our family doctor's voice, modified Groton accent, warm but brisk, following the beep: "Ham Southworth calling to talk to Marv . . . about the radio therapy which *unfortunately* seems *quite* necessary."

In a follow-up call he tells me it will either be a cobalt machine—one-and-a-quarter million volts—or a linear accelerator—six million. I think those are the names, the numbers. All numbers over a thousand have always been the same to me. Whichever, the treatments may or may not make me nauseous. Dr. C., the radiologist, is very meticulous—the best—but not much sense of humor. He should be able to clean up anything Dr. H. might have missed. The prognosis, Dr. Southworth says, is excellent. Sometimes there is a recurrence in five years, but usually this kind remains localized. At worst, as he has already said, it will knock ten years off my life. There is also a hint that if I hadn't made a break for it, the radiation might not have been necessary. No Assisi, no six million volts.

My sister-in-law tells me, if I am nauseous from the radiation, I can smoke marijuana. After a lifetime of conspicuous abstention it would serve me right, the sickly sweet odor floating out from the back bathroom. Daddy and his joints, at it again, the modern equivalent of smoking the reeds from Grandmother Kruidenier's porch chairs in San Diego at age ten, or Iowa corn silk for a twelve-year-old.

5. I think it finally is sinking in that I have had cancer and possibly still do. Dr. Southworth's adverbs "unfortunately" and "quite" outweigh in my memory his adjective, "excellent." Still I don't have—haven't ever had—a symptom to justify the diagnosis or all the activity that has been going on and now promises to continue, whether I believe in it or not.

And all around this nonevent are buttresses being erected by people who obviously have no trouble believing I still have cancer: the doctors and technicians, who aren't, who can't be shocked by the possibility; and, backing them up, the relatives and friends, who probably are shocked just because no loved one is expected to get cancer until, of course, he or she has it, and then the fact sweeps them on—with a certain amount of back-pedaling (a remission is always possible)—to the loved one's death. That is the scenario the past has written. But it never exactly applies. People don't read the proper lines, don't perform the acts as directed. And the audience—I didn't believe, even at the very end, that Tilly or C. were going to die. They might be "dying," but that was different. There was a definite distinction between going to die and "dying." Then, suddenly, there it was: the fact of death.

This is different still—the looking down this particular
tube, this tunnel to one's own death. Having it pointed out,
but not seeing it. The statement "I have cancer"—even, "Marvin has cancer"—lacks conviction. I still don't believe it. And
who knows? Maybe I am right. Maybe it is gone.

6. I do believe it. The suspicion that the doctors don't
know what they are talking about, which has loitered
at the back of my mind since July, has been replaced
with the suspicion that they know more than they are telling
me. Not a sharp suspicion—just a wispy one occupying the
same space.

In this whole sequence, from July till now, no one has
mentioned possible causes for the ulcers, the cancer. I have
mentioned some, and the doctors have permitted my speculations but in no wise confirmed them. The same with the coronary. They come in—all attention, all expertise—to improve
your lot, but again what they do is not presented as a cure, a
complete answer, any more than there was a complete explanation. The patient always seems to be in midstream. I must
admit I am more interested, and have been from the outset,
in the cause than the cure; finding the cause of course implies
a cure, or at least a means of prevention, for others, if not for
oneself.

The final refuge, and reassurance, that there are those
more competent, more understanding than you, if you could
just find them—the ultimate specialist, the definitive clinic—is
an illusion. It is all, in the end, up to you; it is your choice, your
doing, your attempted escape, your responsibility, your deci-

sion, finally, to give space to the answer and, then, if you have time, to pass it along.

January

7. Max, Edna, and Steve came over for New Year's Eve supper, also M.E. Jr. With Irving, this made seven at the table, where the talk was of nuclear holocaust and what you could do about it. I told them all what I thought it would take: prayer, conversion, a critical mass of people suddenly realizing the truth and acting on it, ten just men acknowledging the real purpose of life. No one paid much attention. Why should they? I was neither eloquent, nor coherent, nor loud. And then, with me giving the cue, we fell into a confusion of tongues, a friendly heedlessness with everyone having his say simultaneously.

Max had been given some good news that day concerning his own condition, which had been troubling him for some time. After several CAT scans and a barium enema, his doctors told him that, whatever the problem, it wasn't his cancer that was acting up. Max admitted that the chemotherapy he had received was rough indeed; also, that his interests in life had changed following his various treatments. He didn't say exactly how they had changed, but Max has obviously gentled up, become less hard-edged, although the edge is still there. His is a remarkable performance: writing his column (never missed however sick he was); meeting his academic commitments in San Diego, at Notre Dame; lecturing; and, apparently far advanced in cancer, giving himself his own injections of whatever is his particular poison. Eighty-one.

8. Yesterday I went to my first church service since the operation. They sang "For All the Saints" to the stirring Vaughan Williams tune.

> O blest communion, fellowship divine!
> We feebly struggle, they in glory shine;
> Yet all are one in thee, for all are thine.
> Alleluia! alleluia!

It was one of the three numbers I had scrawled in the back of the red hymnal on the Steinway in the country—just in case. "Sing all the words," I had instructed. "They are worth it."

> And when the strife is fierce, the warfare long,
> Steals on the ear the distant triumph song,
> And hearts are brave again, and arms are strong.
> Alleluia! alleluia!

Although I usually sing out at the cathedral, where there are enough loud voices to cover up my off-key baritone, this time I didn't dare.

9. Last night, for the first time, I dreamt I had cancer. A dream with old friends from Des Moines, whom I hadn't seen in years, showing up for a New York visit, taking one look at me, and knowing, and I knew they knew. Whether it was because of my thinness, my lack of energy, the grayness of my skin, it didn't matter. They knew. There was no question. And that was the worst of all.

* * *

DO your fingernails and toenails drop out in cancer therapy as well as your hair? And if not, why not?

A letter in the morning mail:

> Dear Mr. Barrett;
>
> I am writing to you today to explain why the ongoing cancer research at Memorial Sloan-Kettering is so important to you. Last year in your home state of New York 9,000 died of lung cancer.
> Perhaps someone you know . . . a loved one or a friend. . . .
> Right now there are only 3 ways of treating cancer . . . surgery, treatment using anti-cancer drugs, or radiation. . . .
> But some cancers . . . do not respond well to existing forms of treatment. . . .

10. It is a truism that someone told he has cancer or a serious heart condition suddenly develops a sense of the preciousness of life. I have been told I have both and can't claim any heightening of my perceptions—sensual, spiritual, intellectual, social. What seems to be heightened is memory; not the drowning-man syndrome with your life played backward in a flash, but bits and pieces drifting up, not all necessary pleasant.

* * *

WHAT did Krishna tell Arjuna as he was waiting to go into battle? The words Gerald invoked when I was about to set out for the South Pacific: "Even if thou art the most sinful of all sinners, yet shalt thou cross over all sin by the raft of wisdom. As the burning fire reduces fuel to ashes, O Arjuna, so doth the fire of wisdom reduce all actions to ashes."

Gerald could say it in the words of a half-dozen traditions: "Know thyself." "If the grain dies . . ." Get wise, was what it all boiled down to. How does that stack up against six million volts.

MARY Ellin's stepgrandmother, Anna Case Mackay, has died. Ninety-five years old. Maybe a hundred. No one is sure.

11.

Anna's obituary in the morning *Times:*.

ANNA CASE, A SOPRANO, DEAD:
MADE DEBUT AT THE MET IN '09

Anna Case, a former Metropolitan Opera soprano who sang one of the leading roles, that of Sophie, in the first American production of Richard Strauss's "Der Rosenkavalier" at the Metropolitan Opera House on Dec. 9, 1913, died after a long illness Saturday in her apartment in the Stanhope Hotel in Manhattan.

A picture: "Anna Case in the Vitaphone presentation of 'La Fiesta.'" A white lace mantilla, a Spanish shawl with fringe, a fan, satin pumps. Young, handsome, in charge.

She was never not in charge until suddenly, a year or two ago, there she was: stunned, small, speechless, in her wheelchair in the hotel lobby with her attendant in starched white. That still gave her nine decades of being on the top of things. Four Christmases ago, suddenly joining the carolers in the courtyard of Elizabeth and Alton's apartment building—a pick-up group from a neighborhood church—she silenced them with the strength of her unwavering soprano—"Silent night, holy night"—then swept into the adjacent entry to attend the family feast, leaving them staring in amazement after her.

They are heating the mausoleum in Greenwood Cemetery, cleaning the stained-glass windows for the interment, and sending a car tomorrow to pick us up.

MEANWHILE, upper Broadway, bleak, windblown; a litter of wrappers, bags, containers, whatever it is that is left over when you cook and eat food fast. Babies Hospital is very big, biscuit-colored. Two entrances: the first is barred; a half barricade at the second. A good-looking, sour-faced woman in uniform listens to my question, gives me a sticker to attach to my chest, and points me down the hall and to the left.

It is called the "Radiation Therapy Tunnel" according to the sign on the reception desk. Actually it is the basement below the basement—a windowless warren of offices and rooms, mostly waiting rooms it would seem. The plants are plastic and elaborate, a dead, glossy green. There is an oil painting of kite fliers; a Christmas tree. The people seem less vivid than those I saw four months ago in Dr. H.'s office. Maybe it is familiarity—a common cause. Now we are all in this together.

A young black man in gray trousers and a brown windbreaker is summoned from the waiting room. He is back in less than ten minutes saying, "That is that—for today." Is his "that" what I am going to be having? Coming out, he doesn't look too bad. Not bad at all for having been zapped with six million volts.

NOW I have seen Dr. C., and it is back to square one. Another CAT scan—abdominal—to make sure the spleen, liver, are not involved. A node on the stomach was found to be malignant. I thought there were four. The prognosis is good. Just good. Back to good from excellent. Dr. C. says 35 percent to 50 percent don't have a recurrence. That doesn't sound so good to me. My fingernails won't fall out, not even my hair, but I may be incapacitated for four to five weeks. No guarantee that I will be in shape for "the cancer weekend" the Quakers are holding to support the afflicted at Pendle Hill. Dr. C. wants an oncologist called in—just in case. The horizon broadens. Lymphoma, says Dr. C., is better than plasmacytoma; and anything, everyone agrees, is better than cancer of the stomach. I should be grateful not to have that. So, although I have cancer—or had cancer—*in* the stomach or *around* the stomach, it isn't *of* the stomach. These distinctions are fine and crucial.

WE left *La Bohème* after the third act. Mimi was one of Anna's roles, one she would sing for us in that darkened but still amazing voice, in her shining strapless dress—white shoulders, majestic profile—accompanying herself at the parlor grand. Mimi, Louise, Micaela, Tosca, always winding up with the "Battle Hymn of the Republic": "He has sounded forth the trumpet that shall never call retreat; He is sifting out the hearts of men before his judgment seat. Oh, be swift, my soul, to answer Him! be jubilant, my feet!"

The third act, with its wonderful simulated snow fall, the dark silhouettes moving uphill under their umbrellas, its intimations of worse to come, was sufficient. We didn't wait for the fourth act, for Rodolfo's final, anguished "Mimi." Enough death for one day.

When M.E. and I came out from the opera house the same snow was falling, white, soundless. The first real snow of the winter. We walked under it up Broadway, looking for a cab.

12. I am beginning to feel, since yesterday afternoon, a certain fellowship with other cancer patients. Those gray faces in the tunnel, those still bodies in their wheelchairs, on their stretchers. Will I be so patient, so still. The fear of cowardice is really, I suppose, what the fear of fear is. Of showing it. And if one is willing to be a coward, then isn't that the defeat of fear and the fear behind that and behind that? The diminishing picture of the cereal box on the cereal box on the cereal box finally resolved.

IT is appropriate that radiation therapy should be in a tunnel below a basement—half limbo, half purgatory.

The entrance to the Hotel Umbra in Assisi was a tunnel—
a covered street leading down to the main door—off to the left
a view across roofs to the edge of a valley.

Tunnels on the drive to Urbino, from Siena to Bologna,
between Verona and Salzburg, from Salzburg to Badgastein.

The tunnels on the Amalfi Drive, down the Calabrian
coast, all the way to Sicily.

Tunnels on the Santa Fe and the Southern Pacific all the
way to California through the Rockies, through the Sierras. A
lifetime of tunnels.

Mines and caves are spiritual metaphors. But tunnels are
not, though they should be—from light to light.

The tunnel of love is a joke, not to be taken seriously. A
tunnel isn't sexual. But there it is. We plunge into darkness,
as into the womb, and come out the other end—like birth, like
death. Life, the tunnel.

In mythology I can't think of any tunnels. Caves, mountains, oceans, rivers, but not tunnels. Mazes. Orpheus descend-
ing, leading Euridice up from the underworld. But there was
light at only one end.

The tunnel from prison to freedom: the Count of Monte
Cristo; under the Berlin Wall. The tunnel that comes out into
another prison. Robert Lowell said that the light at the end of
the tunnel was the headlight of an onrushing train. A nasty
thought, but for some reason not a compelling one. We are all
heading in the same direction, even Lowell, who thought he
had turned his back on the light. Behind the locomotive the
light is real, blinding.

The real tunnel goes from light to light. No one would
want to stay in it any longer than necessary.

Necessity determines its length.

13. The 7:15 service at the cathedral. The east of Eden passage from Genesis: "And now art thou cursed from the earth, which hath opened her mouth to receive thy brother's blood from thy hand; When thou tillest the ground, it shall not henceforth yield unto thee her strength; a fugitive and a vagabond shalt thou be in the earth. And Cain said unto the Lord, My punishment is greater than I can bear."

AT ten the limousine picked us up to go to Anna's funeral at St. Patrick's. The second nun from *Dialogues of the Carmelites* sang Schubert's "Ave Maria" and the "Pie Jesu" from Fauré's *Requiem* in the high clear voice, which must have been Anna's at her age.

At Greenwood Cemetery in Brooklyn they unlocked the main gate. Inside there were only a few family members—two black limousinesful—and ten thousand dead, old dead, forgotten dead, under the snow.

Most of the mausoleums are grim little prisons—cells. The Mackays' is something else. Pretty, on its hilltop, a sort of gazebo, a folie, a small rotunda with four sculptures in the gables on four sides. Inside, a mosaic floor, a domed ceiling of tile, a white marble madonna. The stained-glass windows are of the beatitudes.

Outside, from the porch, one can see the cold, clean silhouette of lower Manhattan.

The talk on the ride back and over a delicious lunch in a small, noisy, East Side restaurant was all of where one would like to be buried.

14. A visit to Oz to discuss my future. He insists, with his customary optimism and kindness, that I stay on, that a simple gastrectomy is no reason to retire before my time. "Stay on and we'll see." Meanwhile, the trustees in Jacksonville are restless. They want a meeting to discuss "things," which means trouble.

15. M., M.E., and I went to hear Bernstein conduct the Mahler *Resurrection Symphony*. There was wild applause—the whole house on its feet and Bernstein lurching about the platform embracing people, a Silenus in evening dress. Not old, just ravaged.

I would prefer Mahler to be coherent, but, if he were, perhaps the music would be too much to bear. The final movement was upsetting enough as it was: a huge orchestra, a huge chorus, Jessye Norman (huge) singing at the top of her huge voice:

> With wings I have won for myself
> I shall soar in fervent love aloft
> To the light no eye has yet beheld!
> I shall die to live again!
> Thou shalt rise again, yes again, my heart
> in a single moment!
> The battle's brave heartbeat
> Will bear thee up to God.

Mahler wrote the words and music when he was thirty-five and died when he was fifty.

Dying is no longer something someone else does.

It never was.

16. Perhaps, after all, if it persists, the cancer will be the means of my getting control of my own life. For almost as long as I can remember my behavior has been a matter of action and reaction, someone's else action, me never taking the truly creative step—always answering, never questioning. This could be my chance at some sort of freedom. I seem to sense an opening, and the fact that it is limited in time is of no consequence, indeed, is meaningless. That it exists and that I go through it are the important things. This must be the new view of space and time that my fellow victims speak of, that a few days back I denied having experienced.

17. What appeared to be a tunnel, or what I declared a tunnel or imagined a tunnel—a thing with light at both ends—has, it seems, gone dark behind, ahead, as though suddenly it were bending or sagging, which I guess is a possibility. A bendable tunnel, flexible, so that the light comes and goes according to your disposition—heavy, devious—a highly sensitive tube, but still a tube, all middle, dark or otherwise, until the end.

18. I have been noticing lately the difference between reading newspapers and magazines and reading books. I can tolerate journalism best in the morning and midday, but as the day proceeds, journals become more irritating and difficult to assimilate, simply by virtue of their relation to time—their episodic and transitory nature. From noon on, books are much preferred. They represent security, repose, duration in time and space, something substantial to rest on. The reassurance comes not from what the words say, but from their number: this is substantial company; I can lose myself in it. I notice this particular advantage disappears as I approach the end of a book. Then the nervousness, the irritability reasserts itself. The end is in sight, and the world and its concerns, which the papers and magazines represent, are there waiting.

A book is a tunnel.

COMPUTERIZED Tomography, where CAT scans are given, is on the third floor of Columbia Presbyterian, at least five floors above the tunnel. You wait in a wide place in the corridor. It is a battle zone. The wall behind you has been blown out. There is a litter of large cardboard boxes. Oxygen tanks are strewn about. The ceiling is being torn away. There is an old man strapped to a stretcher. A grizzled man in a porkpie hat is drinking orange liquid from a big paper cup.

The receptionist has never heard of me. Where is my requisition? She goes away without waiting for an answer. She comes back; gives me a stern look. I must return to Babies Hospital and pay my money up front.

But the Babies Hospital cashier has closed her window. I can see her back there. I rap on the glass, but she does not attend to my signal.

Now I am twentieth in line at the clinic cashier. This is the line for poor people who have to wait for requisitions for medicine and transportation. I obviously don't belong here, the cashier tells me. I should go to Mrs. Enright. Mrs. Enright sends me to Central Registration. No one wants my money after four.

Now I am going to Vanderbilt; down the hall—that hall, the lady points—they'll take my money. Rose will help me. Fifty minutes later I pay my $158 and get a receipt and return to the CAT scan waiting area.

The man in the porkpie hat has drunk his plastic container of orange drink. The receptionist says good night to me and to the man in the porkpie hat and a big fellow in a plaid wrapper in a wheelchair. Someone, she tells me, is researching my appointment.

I have a little fit. They are running forty-five minutes late, she admits. She gives me a big cup of apple juice to shut me up. I should drink a cup every ten minutes. The gentleman in the porkpie hat tells me he has been waiting since one. He is a retired butcher who now works with horses—pacers and trotters—at Yonkers and Roosevelt raceways. He has a bad back.

It is now 6:20. A pleasant lady in a smock comes out to say that the patient in the plaid wrapper is going directly to the operating room. Two big guys in blue coveralls take him away. The man in the porkpie hat is up. I'm next. I should be out by eight.

Don't go to the bathroom, she tells me. A full bladder is desirable. The discomfort—acute—begins.

Finally I am in the room with the big object: a collar that becomes a tunnel when they push me into it. A flashing light, a roar, a beep, and I can breathe until the next time. Thirty-five flashes and I am through.

After all that—the pleasant lady in the smock who is in charge—says the pictures look fine, but she can't say for sure, of course.

Of course.

19. Dr. Southworth confirmed that a negative CAT scan report would not alter the therapy plan. (I am obviously still hoping for the positive intrusion—the simple statement: "Enough, no more.") He said nothing smaller than a marble shows up on the scan anyway. There may still be some pea-sized objects floating around in my midriff—bean-sized; bead-sized; the size of those small clay marbles they used in important competitions when I was in grammar school, arranged in a cross at the center of a big circle in the sandlot out behind Perkins Elementary. Clay marbles or pea-sized objects, they must be shot out before you win, before they begin to split and spread.

A long, involved dream in which I am trapped in a fatal predicament: a shingle of loose shale crumbling under me and, at the bottom of the slope, a precipice. People are shouting encouragement as I slip. I wake.

Somewhere in the dream someone was described as having lymphoma and being "wonderful," although she knew that she was dying. I said to myself, "I have lymphoma too."

The important thing about the dream, however, was my getting out of it. I had landed myself in an impossible, a deadly spot. There was no escape—except to wake up. Death or waking—the fact that I still have the choice is the encouraging thing. I can still wake up. I still want to wake up. I don't want to go back, lose my footing, and slide down that crumbling, seductive slope to destruction, no matter how much my companions admire me for having gotten so far in an impossible direction. They remain in the dream. I wake.

Of course, another way to look at it is that dying and waking up are the same thing, or seem to be. We seem to be dying, and we are only waking up; we seem to be waking up, and we are only dying.

The revelation came not from the dream itself, but from the mechanics of dreaming, of getting out of the dream—the symbol of dreaming and waking; not one or the other, but the borderline between.

My waking life parallels this dream. I am working myself into an increasingly impossible position—inching forward into the inescapable, the unsurvivable impasse—to the point where the choice is death or waking.

In life I have a few times given myself the illusion of escape without really waking. But it is only an illusion, and the process of entanglement, of involvement—illusion itself—continues, and one by one the footholds disappear and in front of me—forward or back—there remains that simple choice: death or waking. But is it a choice?

20. It is beautiful out: a white clinging snow
I read the Tower of Babel story at the service this morning. God the troublemaker. Henry Robinson Luce on high.

THIS evening, the weekly group at the Gurdjieff Foundation. Sixteen years of meetings. These are old friends, and I have yet to learn half their names. Gurdjieff may not be exactly my style—too ornery, too hard-boiled—but still I have hung on. These are people who care about the noumenal—as Gerald would say—not the phenomenal; the spirit, not the flesh; the reality, not the appearance. They don't look different: no better nor worse dressed; no uglier nor prettier than any other group gathered for a serious purpose. Lord P., the stand-in for Gerald decades later, is taller, thinner, with less hair. Another upper class Briton, beautifully educated, the right accent, kindly disposed, born in the faith but obdurately heterodox. Still, like Gerald, pointing me back to where he came from. Someone, again, whom I can admit knows more, much more, than I and is willing to pass at least some of his knowledge along. The resemblance, quite remarkable when I think of it, ends there.

I asked Lord P. about death. In all the years I have known him, have attended these meetings, death has not come up. He spoke carefully and quietly. I heard every word, took exception to none, and then forgot the lot.

How little I remember of these crucial questions and answers. A lifetime of telling observations, words of wisdom lost or misplaced. More preserved from Gerald than most, but when you think of all those letters, all those conversations, it amounts to bits and pieces: "There is no chance nor accident; all is meaning and design." "The opposable thumb." "Integral thought." "A working hypothesis." "The union of all who pray and who by prayer grow in love and understanding may yet prove to be the basis of that universal church which is mankind's hope."

Aldous in the kitchen at Trabuco telling us about the possessed Sisters of Loudun, Grandier, the spoiled priest, the saintly Father Surin, as we washed up after tea. Aldous on the sofa in Tilly's tiny living room talking about Trabuco, the community's collapse: "It was all too sad. Too unutterably sad." The "unutterably" pronounced as only Aldous could pronounce it, with such delicacy, such conviction. I can still hear that voice rising up to the treble, sliding back to the diapason, one word stretched to its limit. But why, indeed, did that seventeenth-century congregation of high-powered French Catholics, as well as our pathetic little California commune, have to turn out badly? The answer is lost.

Another voice: Mother Theresa in our dilapidated Volkswagon. As reward for giving her Missionaries of Charity an afternoon a month I had her with me all the way from the convent in the South Bronx to Pennsylvania Station, and what did she say? What hints by which I might better dispose my life? The splendid, burnt-out buildings we drove by—wasted when they might have housed the homeless. The derelicts on the sidewalks. "The poor of New York are in much more pain than the poor of Calcutta. Sourer, more hopeless." The message was simple but still beyond my capabilities.

And what had I gleaned from Krishnamurti the two times when, once out of curiosity, once from distress, I had sought him out. "There is no need for an authority, a guru, a god, a church." Just that? Nothing else? I balked.

And what about all those trivial questions I as a journalist was expected to ask, hastily conceived, the answers half attended to while I formulated my next question—most not worth attention anyway. The canned responses of the rich and famous: virtuosi, novelists, painters, movie kings and queens. Nothing to do with their real lives, their real thoughts, doubts, dreads. The delible album of the hack. A wicked waste of time, of paper. The Tower of Babel indeed.

21. Yesterday I ran into Marge B. on the stairs. She asked me how I was. I told her I was about to go into radiation. She said they had Dick put an ice bag on his head when they gave him chemotherapy so his hair wouldn't fall out. He pushed it off saying he had always wanted to be bald. I asked Marge if Dick's hair had indeed fallen out. She said there hadn't been time.

MY mother-in-law called. In the course of the conversation my CAT scan was mentioned, and she told me that she had never approved of CAT scans because of the research done at the American Museum of Natural History on live cats and she felt this was a bad thing for children who might hear that such things were happening to friendly animals. Three more stories, beginning with one about little M.E., who in the same museum had been distressed to see all the dead animals. Who were the mean people who had killed them? Mrs. B. had looked at the plaques with the donors' names and was able to assure M.E. that the donors were all dead too. And not even stuffed.

Which led to the story about big M.E. requesting an all black outfit for her grandfather's funeral and, when she was refused, saying petulantly, "You are spoiling all my fun." And finally to her granddaughter Rachel, who told her grandmother that she liked funerals and would enjoy going to hers and, of course—not wishing to play favorites—to those of all her other grandparents as well.

The conversation ended with her suggestion that I not tell my friends that I had cancer since I would always be getting unwanted and upsetting advice and information about my affliction. Just say it is your heart that is causing all the trouble, she advised, since everyone already knows about that and you won't stir up additional sympathy and concern.

*   *   *

MORE cancer talk at a dinner party, my first since the operation. Everyone tells me how well I look, avoiding my eyes. Maybe Mrs. B. is right. But then the talk turned to Martha S., whom I first knew as a leggy ten-year-old playing hopscotch on her front walk in Des Moines while I was inside being encouraged by her father to apply for a scholarship to Harvard. (So I was six months late in sending in the forms. Maybe something could be worked out without taking the college boards. It had been.) Martha had reappeared a lifetime later as a handsome middle-aged woman on crutches at a Du Pont Awards ceremony, a distinguished producer of TV documentaries, very sick, cured, then sick again. I went to see her not too long ago. Hair cropped, thin, the remission apparently over, she was in her pullman kitchen preparing a gourmet lunch for the two of us. Talk about what I owed her family, the state of the world, the decline of TV journalism. And now I am told she is cured yet again by some miracle worker in Germany, a new technique. I must call her and find out about it. Just in case.

A carcinogen story in the morning *Times:* EDB, a chemical prevalent in grains and citrus crops. A lifetime use, the article says, could be responsible for cancer in three out of a thousand of the population. Could I be one of the unlucky three? All that orange juice. All that whole wheat bread.

22. In the five months since I was told I had cancer, I don't believe I have said, "I've got cancer" once, in so many words, to myself or to anyone else, although one way or another people get the idea. Still, however much I want them to know, it is a very hard thing to say straight out. Similar in some strange way to the AA's saying, "I am an alcoholic." And, of course, now my hope is that I no longer have it, that it has been taken from me, lifted out. But does one have to acknowledge, as the alcoholics do, that having once had it, it is a permanent condition? Once an alcoholic, always an alcoholic. Is the analogy that complete?

This all came up when I began considering the advisability of calling Martha S. and asking her for information about her German cure and indeed about the whole course of her disease, one cancer patient to another. There was no reason she should know that I was one too.

And then, at the cathedral, as I headed for coffee and cookies after the service, there she stood—Martha looking glorious in her black fur coat and hat, and boots. It was one of those minor miracles which some people call coincidence. I had made up my mind to phone her about Germany that afternoon. But it wasn't Germany. It was Italy, Lake Como. And it was not a complete cure, but building up your immune system. So I had cancer. So what else was new? Join the club. Not that flip, but at least no alarm or horror at the news. Call her tomorrow and she'd give me a list of the diet supplements I should take. A doctor is very important—one you can talk to who is sympathetic, i.e., on your wave length, not sympathetic, boohoo. The same thing that Max said. The meeting gave me a real boost, and she didn't bother to say I was looking great.

AS I arrived back at the apartment, the phone rang. It was a friend calling to say that Jerry Toobin, in charge of my broadcast at Channel 13, had died. A fiercely sweet, civilized man, and his brain tumor had been benign.

23. I am back in the therapy tunnel to have my "block" made. A new meaning for a word that already has too many. Block to play with, the block you live on, block that kick! the block that Mary Queen of Scots, and Anne Boleyn and Saint Thomas More died on. And now a block to keep the radiation from going where it shouldn't go.

DR. C. comes into a small room dominated by a big, pale green x-ray machine and tells me to strip to the waist. Dr. I., a young Argentine with rimless glasses, assists him. The x-ray machine has a place for me to lie on and stare up at a square aperture. They lower me, raise me, shift me from side to side, give me a half cup of barium to drink, take pictures, measure me with calipers. A fellow with fly-away blond hair beginning halfway back his scalp comes in and lays a metal strip between my armpits. Dr. C. and Dr. I. stick me with bits of tape, then draw X's and lines on my chest. It all takes a little more than an hour.

HANDEL'S *Rinaldo* at the Met from Anna's box. Marilyn Horne as a Christian commander in a horsehair helmet and brass breastplate. A bunch of tumblers from New Jersey turning the battle scene into a spectacular vaudeville act. Wonderful music. A happy ending. Would that all wars could be transformed from horror and boredom to pure entertainment.

* * *

THE area marked for radiation—a crude square in blood red indelible ink with a target mark, a circle with an X at the center—is much higher than I expected, missing the area where I think my stomach is. Above, to the left, over my heart.

24. What is the word for "sock" in Italian? In French? Should I have oatmeal or Nutri-Grain for breakfast? Should I go to Darjeeling or the Grand Canyon once I'm through with my radiation therapy? The world's biggest heap or its biggest (visible) hole? What are the questions I should ask Dr. O, the oncologist, today. How will I know if the lymphoma is recurring, when it was only a fluke that they found it in the first place? What about my chest? What will the radiation do to my immune system? What about x-rays from now on? Should I avoid them since I am going to develop this intimate relationship with a ten-billion-volt machine? How many roentgens does that add up to?

A half hour's prayers shot to hell. Forty years since I began to pray, and that is the best I can do.

A visit to Dr. O., Department of Oncology, Columbia Presbyterian Hospital.

The visit is encouraging. It is also expensive: $250 for a brief examination, a few minutes talk, not including the B_{12} shot I get on my way out. Dr. O., young, serious, dark-haired, had no recommendation for chemotherapy, although that obviously is where he makes his big bucks. An 80 percent chance of no recurrence, with the odds building year by year to 100 percent if no recurrence after five years. The vitamin B_{12} shot is to avoid pernicious anemia, since the part of the stomach that assimilates that vitamin has been eliminated. I'll need one a month for the rest of my life. Dr. O. emphasized the rest of my life aspect of my affliction. The same as with the heart, I'll never be off the hook. His odds are much better than Dr. C.'s

NOW I am back in the tunnel waiting room. There are three stretchers out by the nurses' desk. Three men—two older, one younger than myself—are in the room with me. The younger man, wearing pale corduroy trousers and a heavy, dark red sweater, has lost his hair and is flushed. I can see the X on his skull. One of the stretcher cases—comatose, with two IV's and three attendants—was just wheeled out.

An older man in a black-and-white plaid flannel shirt has come in and crossed the waiting room to the men's room. He has deep magenta markings across his jaw and neck and around the back of his head.

A stretcher goes by with a young woman with corn-colored hair and a purple silk blouse.

Now a man with X's and a week's growth of beard on his jaws—the aspect of the classic hobo, the homeless bum, the old prospector after a fruitless winter in the hills—a shuffling walk—he could be sixty, younger, older, who can tell—slouches into the chair opposite. Whatever he once was, he obviously no longer is.

I am now on it, under it: a larger, newer, shinier machine in a big low-ceilinged room. Alongside me is a six-foot photo-mural of a beach and sea. There is a small rectangular hole chipped into the waves. O. (brunette) and B. (blond) have slipped me into the machine's jaws and are adjusting me up, down, sideways. Above me there is a black square hole that grows smaller and larger on command. There are diagonal thread marks across the hole. I am the target.

First they take pictures. Then they zap me: ninety rads on the front; ninety rads on the back. The machine rolls over. I lay still. Very still. It isn't cobalt. It is a linear accelerator, whatever that means.

I get up, put on my Johnny coat backwards without tying the strings. An old gentleman in a blue dressing gown in a wheelchair is waiting by the monitors for his turn. I smile. He doesn't smile back; just looks at my stomach where the marks are.

THE fourth floor above the Doubleday Bookstore at Fifty-third and Fifth. A comfortable, make-believe flat expensively decorated. They all are there for this publication party: the friends and acquaintances of the author, a poet who has written a biography of a poet. It could be the Hamptons except for Fifth Avenue and a cold foggy drizzle outside. I float through the crowd, meeting the searching glances directly—a balloon bouncing sideways toward the buffet, only I am no balloon. I have lost twenty pounds since most of these people last saw me. But I don't need propping up, although half the people there look at me as though they'd like to do something to help. Mary Ellin finally steers me back through the crowd, no better nor worse than when I arrived.

25. A morning at the office screening cancer films deliberately chosen from all the other entries. A Hodgkins disease victim and his family. A little boy whose hair fell out from radiation therapy. "One out of four will die of cancer." "The majority of cancers can be cured." Terry Drinkwater tells about his cancer of the throat on the "Today Show." There is *my* CAT scan machine, *my* linear accelerator!

There are, I am told, other cures less damaging to the body, less risky, than radiation and chemotherapy—biological ones. I wonder why I am not being given those. One tape stresses the importance of the team approach. No team for me; just one doctor after another.

I tell Janet that, thanks to the tapes she had picked out for me to view, I am beginning to consider cancer a second-rate, easily curable, vulgar disease—no big deal—But maybe it is too much TV viewing—low-level radiation, that has caused my condition.

DO you suppose it was stubbornness that did it? Stubbornness about my writing—sticking to it despite all the nasty editors, the inattentive readers, the indifferent critics. Stubbornness about my job—ignoring the eager kibitzers, the outraged executives, plugging ahead. Stubbornness about my marriage—overcoming the initial uncertainties, the continuing challenges and adjustments (thirty years of them), never thinking of giving up. Enough to give anyone a stomachache. I am still asking the question "where does it come from?" as though the cancer might be coming back, terminal or worse. "Terminal" seems to be the operative word. At any rate, the ache is there. I presume because of the Big Machine—the obvious explanation.

* * *

LAST night I talked to M.—the first time I had seen her since *Dialogues of the Carmelites*—about our disease as a death warrant. Things have changed, we agreed. Cancer no longer equals certain death, and yet, although we know this to be clinically true, neither of us, inside, is convinced. We have been so conditioned to think otherwise, have seen so many others die with cancer to blame. Still, the odds improve daily, and something else, some other dread disease may soon be taking cancer's place as the number one certain killer (heart disease doesn't count, I tell myself), perhaps already has.

As for her secret, she has shared it with only two or three friends. She keeps it to herself, she says with spirit, because she doesn't want sympathy, doesn't want gossip, doesn't want people to say she has had an easy life, had everything her way, and now, the woman who has everything, has cancer. Fair enough.

And then I tried to explain why I felt impelled to tell everyone now that there is no question of my any longer avoiding the fact. If not straight out, at least by implication, so that there would be no question of the truth. I do this not in hope of sympathy, but as a provocation, a defiance, perhaps even a punishment for others not so afflicted. What do all of you jokers make of this piece of information, this nasty bit of news? But more than that, it is a way of facing the truth myself—What, after all, does it mean?—and perhaps forcing other people to face the truth as well. I don't know that I have succeeded in this missionary purpose, even in a small way. But once the message has been delivered—directly, indirectly—I don't feel at all timid; indeed, it gives me a feeling of power. I have it, the worst supposedly has happened, and it isn't all that bad. *You* can still dread it.

Although if what M. and I say to reassure each other (forget about all the rest), if what we have been discussing is true, then my advantage will be lost along with the reason for her to keep her secret. We will rejoin the great undifferentiated mass of people who are a little more sick than well. Cancer—what is so great about that? Fading into oblivion with polio, TB, diphtheria, leprosy, the Black Death.

Upon consideration, M.'s reasons for telling nothing and mine for telling all seem equally misguided.

26. Read the lesson from Acts at the service this morning. Paul on the road to Damascus. The blinding flash. The voice saying, "Saul, Saul. Why persecutest thou me?" Where would we all be if Saul hadn't fallen off his horse?

A letter:

> Dear Dr. C.,
>
>   Thank you very much for your kind referral of Mr. Barrett, whom I had the pleasure of seeing in my office on January 24, 1984. As you know, he is a very nice gentleman who underwent a partial gastrectomy on December 12, 1983, by Dr. H. for a gastric lymphoma with pathology revealing well-differentiated lymphocytic lymphoma. He apparently had no evidence of disease elsewhere observed at surgery and had previously been evaluated at St. Luke's Hospital where CAT scan and bone-marrow biopsy as well as

chest x-ray and routine chemistries were all within normal limits.

At the time that I saw him he was regaining weight lost during the surgical period. He denied any fever, chills, sweats, and had no specific pulmonary, gastrointestinal, urologic, or other symptoms to suggest disease elsewhere. On physical exam he was a healthy-appearing 63-year-old with normal vital signs, no adenopathy, no liver or spleen enlargement, normal heart with clear lungs but with decreased breath sounds.

I discussed with him and his wife the various options available. I indicated that radiotherapy under your supervision was clearly needed to supplement his surgery and increase chances for a cure. It seemed to me that chemotherapy was not really indicated at this time. Although it did offer the possibility of eradicating any microscopic deposits of lymphoma elsewhere. His lack of disease elsewhere and the relatively good prognosis histology of his lymphoma suggested that his chances for cure were quite reasonable without chemotherapy. He himself was clearly not in favor of a program of chemotherapy, realizing that it did offer the possibility of decreasing the risk of recurrence but the disadvantage of having to undergo whatever toxicity was associated with it. I would add that most oncologists now feel that isolated gastric lymphomas with this histology do not require adjuvant chemotherapy after radiotherapy.

I also suggested to him that because of his gastrectomy he receive B-12 injections periodically and indeed gave him one that day. He is always welcome to come to my office for those, but I suspect it will be easier for him to receive them either at the Columbia campus or with Dr. S.

He is a very pleasant man who hopefully has a very good prognosis. I will be available should any problems arise where I can be of help.

Thank you once again for asking me to participate in his care.

Sincerely yours,

"Microscopic deposits of lymphoma"? "Decreased breath sounds"? *Relatively* good"? "A very pleasant man who *hopefully* (italics mine) has a very good prognosis"?

My sweats (cold) were my own business; had nothing, so far as I could see, to do with him.

AT breakfast Mary Ellin hugged me and said, "You know you are going to get well." My instant response was, "I never have considered for a minute that I wouldn't." Not quite true. But then not completely false either.

27. I am arriving earlier and earlier at the tunnel—before eight this morning. A middle-aged woman I have seen before got into the elevator, coughing. "Asthma," she said with a soft Spanish accent; also, "Tired, tired." "The radiation?" I say. She nods. She is wearing a brown coat and black cotton kerchief on her head. "The radiation. Here."

Two times she gestures toward her armpit. "Not here," toward her breast. She looks tired.

THERE are four African violets under a violet light next to the sink in the radiation room. Very healthy. Opposite are the blocks: ninety or one hundred ungainly chunks of lead— cubes, bent rectangles; odd, thick, misshapen. Dr. C. has decided I don't need one. Red ink is enough. No additional protection necessary. The lead lumps are for those who really belong here.

I lie on my steel tray. For thirty seconds nothing happens. Then for another thirty seconds nothing happens again. The invisible confronting the invisible. The atoms in my belly being bombarded by the atoms that the linear activator shoots at me, although they really don't know that there is anything in there for them to hit, to knock out. The beyond-Star-Wars aspect of the whole exercise. It is odd that the place designated for bombardment is even closer to the seat of prayer, as I envision it, than the gastrectomy. Will six million volts affect my soul? The *scintilla dei* hit and extinguished. Or will it be like the Russian astronauts who decided they had disproved the existence of God and his heaven when they didn't run into either of them "up there." Nothing but sky. Nothing but skin and guts.

28. Woke at 4:00 A.M., turned on the lamp. Above it were the engravings of Taormina as it was in the eighteenth century, as it still was in 1953 when we lived there for the winter. Castelmola on its pinnacle, Fontana Vecchia on the far side of the deep, brush-filled ravine. Two of the views from the garden of our four-room, unheated casa; another, down through the fingers of cypress, across the campo santo, and on beyond to Ulysses' wine-dark Ionian Sea. The bray of donkeys, chickens, a Vespa roaring up the hill on an invisible road. Memory at work again.

On the wall behind me is Sheila Isham's wash of the fields of Sagaponack—over the pillows and faraway. Another outlook, this one from our white farmhouse within the sound of the northern sea—a line of dunes across an open meadow, a gray sky. A house filled with children and guests. At night, the pound of the waves. Was the heart already damaged? The cancer long since sown?

ON the way to lunch at Martha S.'s on Bank Street I went through another of our old neighborhoods. New York is filled with them, some more recognizable than others. At first glance, this one, the West Village, seemed little changed. Looking closer, there was now a hairdresser instead of One Two Kangaroo, where we used to buy the children's birthday and Christmas, Valentine, and Easter presents. The Loews, where Irving and I went to a matinee of *Doctor Zhivago* when he was nine, a bleak afternoon, both of us upset by that long and hopeless story—the old man struck down within sight of his long lost love—the Loews was gone, and the big tangled community garden that replaced it as well. Now there was a parking lot for heavy equipment. The Italian grocery store was a Parisian patisserie—very chic, glass brick, black-and-white checks. The pharmacy long since had given way to an Aspen-style restaurant—soups and salads. The little Greek temple of St. John's in the Village, destroyed by a fire, was now all brick and stained glass. John Cannon, the rector, was standing out front in his shirt sleeves. He took me into the garden where I used to sit in the sun outside the apartment we rented on the close, reading the Sunday morning papers, waiting for the children to return from church school. The grown-ups didn't go to church in those days. "We're selling off the houses one by one," John said, "but special covenants preserve the garden. They can't cut it up or build out into it."

MARTHA receives me in her bedroom, big, facing south across a garden with sun streaming in, filled with the trophies of her trips—to India, Java, China, Japan, Russia, Samarkand. She is propped up with a mountain of colorful pillows behind her, looking pretty but obviously in pain, trying hard to find a comfortable position, talking to me all the while about my cancer, about hers, about everybody's. About alternate therapies, about diet, about surgery, radiation, chemo; she has had them all.

After twenty years in this house, she is going to have to move. Find something new. Being put out.

She gives me some chicken soup sent by her friends who run an experimental community up on Cape Cod. The latest in subsistence farms—the chain of life respected. A new approach and hope. Good soup. Good bread. Good salad. She tells me that the Simontons have split up. LeShan is no longer working with cancer victims; burnt out. But Kübler-Ross, who was having a hard time—how long can you stare down death?—has been rehabilitated by the Quakers at their community at Pendle Hill. We talk a little about Pendle Hill; my plan to go there for a cancer weekend. Why not? It can't hurt. It may even help.

She tells me about the cancer support group she used to belong to. Maybe I'd like to start one. She withdraws the suggestion. Not such a good idea. There were always one or two negative presences dragging the others down, and eventually, when one of the members died, as was inevitable, the group flew apart, couldn't stand up to the loss. So what was the use? The whole purpose of coming together gone at the critical moment, subverted.

How would I feel if one of my team, my crew, should die, go into a decline while I looked on, giving up the ghost, deserting me, breaking the chain? I really don't know. I watched both Tilly and C. go, slowly, irreversibly slipping over the edge. But that was different. The difference is that then I wasn't yet one of them.

I look at Martha rearranging her pillows, trying to get into a comfortable position, not succeeding. "It isn't, thank God, cancer again," she tells me. "It is just this condition in my back." "Who needs it?" I respond. "After what you've been through, who needs it?"

I pretend to believe her. Force myself to believe her. The third cure *had* worked. She was the seasoned veteran; I, the raw recruit.

"I'll see you at the awards," I say.

She smiles a suddenly wan smile and nods.

"Without fail."

"Without fail."

Pendle Hill

February

1. Pendle Hill: A Quaker Center for Study and Contemplation, Wallingford, Pa.

To: Participants in THE CHALLENGE OF CANCER, February 3–5

Dear Friends:

Greetings from a snowy Pendle Hill and from Irene, Kitty and Howard. We are all looking forward to having you with us for the weekend beginning February 3. A couple of reminders: bring comfortable, casual clothing. We are an informal kind of place and sitting on the floor in front of the fireplace, walking in the woods, and exploring the campus may be things you wish to include in your free time. Also, as mentioned on the enclosed schedule, you are invited to bring copies of brief readings, excerpts, or music that you may wish to share.

THE less than half a man on a skateboard is on the subway shaking his can at me and saying, "Thank you." No "God bless you" or "Have a good day" from him. A black man in stretch leather hanging on a strap, lots of studs and an earring, bends low to make his contribution, green and folding.

PENNSYLVANIA Station. I haven't been here since I came with the Missionaries of Charity, lugging a coffee urn and boxes of sandwiches for the bag ladies and derelicts in my antique messenger's outfit, scruffy windbreaker, and baggy trousers. We'd just been bounced, all of us, sisters and coworkers alike, thrown out of Grand Central by the police, who told us we were encouraging the homeless. Pennsylvania Station was much more hospitable. And then suddenly across the waiting room was B.—a Harvard golden boy, barely tarnished, on his way to some palace in New Jersey—spotting me at the same time as I spotted him. Our eyes locked. His said, "What in God's name is *he* doing with all those bums and ladies in blue-and-white saris? Is he getting himself a free coffee and handout? Has it come to that? Harvard Class of '42?" He didn't come over to see. Better not to know.

Better not to know this time as well. On my way to "A Cancer Weekend" and "A Quaker Retreat." Although my clothes were a little smarter, and I wasn't consorting with bums and bag ladies and women in saris.

7:30–8:30 P.M. Waysmeet Living Room

> Howard R. will lead us with our introductions: Who are you? Why did you come? What is your main interest in the subject? What do you want to discuss mostly?

Howard R. Big, hearty man. Not sick looking at all. One of three leaders. Starts us out. First contact with the disease was seeing his favorite uncle die of cancer of prostate after fighting two years. His brother-in-law died after four years. Five years ago told to look into his own prostate. Ignored advice for two years. Told he had malignant tumor and should start radiation therapy. Decided on alternative methods three years ago— rejected radiation. Doing diet, meditation, etc. Cancer has made him more spiritually aware.

Angelica E. Mother, two sisters died of cancer. Found out just before Christmas she had it. Offered radiation versus surgery. Now, in fourth week of recovery.

Mary H. Young woman, red-haired, big, healthy looking. Two grandfathers died of cancer, one grandmother, two cousins. Day before her thirtieth birthday (she looks twenty) told she had level-four melanoma of the leg. Visualization therapy for two weeks before operation. No other kind of therapy.

Martin C. Completed radiation therapy eight days ago. Looks frail, beat. Lost his hair. First diagnosed as epileptic. Negative CAT scan ruled out tumor; now CAT scan is positive. Dangerous primary tumor. Heard tumor of brain rather easily beaten by radiation therapy. Came from Britain in 1961. Feels committed to ordinary American treatment—didn't want to be too esoteric.

Barbara L. Problems began eleven years ago. Leg and intestines. Allergic to certain smells. Doctors told her it was in her mind. Ended in homeopathic clinic in Chicago. Joined a natural foods group. Discovered cancer. Had radiation. Friends told her she must have natural treatment. Went to Germany on crutches. Nutritional treatment helped other leg. Stress. Finding help wherever she could. Went to psychics, etc.

Tom J. Lifetime of good health. Active athlete. Olympics competitor. One and a half years ago had physical before leaving country; referred to urologist; had three operations in ten days. Prostate cancer. Six weeks of daily cobalt radiation. Now chemotherapy.

Ginny R. Is in midst of recurrence of cancer that started five years ago. Hysterectomy, chemotherapy; told she was cured. After five years found tumor on her ribs. Had chemotherapy. Decided to do macrobiotic diet. Did it for two months. Didn't like dietician. After two months, spots on her lungs. Gave up diet. Chemotherapy has been changed. Now has tumors on her legs. Everything is on hold right now.

Kitty B. Husband got cancer in '76, recurrence in '79. Found copy of a LeShan book in a health food store. Tried to get husband interested. He was more comfortable with traditional medicine. Died at their summer place two years ago. Three children—fourteen, seventeen, and nineteen.

Rosaleen Q. Breast cancer. Radical mastectomy. Told to have chemotherapy. She refused. Wanted to read books. Told books just make trouble. Demanded another oncologist who gave her five-drug chemotherapy. Bad reaction to one drug. In chemotherapy for a year. Did research on all drugs. Went to the Simonton's workshop. Discovered that Compazine, one of the drugs, had yellow dye number three in it—a carcinogen. Protected her body as best she could. Now two years.

Shirley O. Three years ago her brother-in-law had cancer of colon; was operated on. A year ago her father discovered cancer of prostate; was operated on. A year later chemotherapy recommended. Several prayer groups pray for her father each time he gets chemotherapy. Here to learn how to be helpful.

Lorna M. A year ago last fall told she had a hernia. Turned out to be cancer. Surgeon said he got it all out except for a few specks—twelve treatments then they'll open her up again. "I wept about my hair. I didn't weep about anything else."

Morris M. Lorna's husband. Two sisters died of cancer. Thirteen months ago when Lorna learned she had it, Morris built her a swimming pool.

Tom D. Three years ago Saint Valentine's Day found out about it. Never smoked. Never drank. Blood test every two months. Three trips to Ceylon and India. On last trip bothered by constipation; got worse. Operated on in hospital in Colombo. Brilliant operation. Not shocked by news he had cancer at all. Wife told him. Already past seventy when he was told. Surgeon explained how he took his lower colon out and then put it back in. He was carried to operating room on a canvas stretcher, felt enveloped in calmness. Stayed on from February to April. Almost died of Asian flu. Had chemotherapy after he got home.

Irene C. Trying to live a stress-free life here on the staff at Pendle Hill and trying to get well through alternate therapies, visualization—the Simonton's scheme for making the good cells stare down the bad.

Marvin B. Nothing about his flirtation with alternate means. Considerable about his shock at getting cancer after thinking he had taken care of his particular track to the hereafter with heart disease. A muddled comment on the psychic origins of it all. Nothing about Assisi. Half way through radiation therapy. They think they've got it all.

8:30–9:00 P.M. Donald Swann will play the piano for us. Sing or listen, as you feel inclined.

Swann told us that his mother dying of cancer when he was thirteen was what turned him to a career in music. He played a bit, then led us in "Kum Ba Yah," "Lord of the Dance," "Mother Teresa's Prayer," and something of his own composition, I believe, called the "Hippopotamus Song":

> Mud, mud, glorious mud
> Nothing quite like it for cooling the blood
> So follow me, follow
> Down to the hollow
> And there let us wallow
> In glorious mud.

2. Last night, listening to the testimonies, one wondered at the actual difference between the so-called legitimate treatments for cancer and the alternative ones. How much of the psychological-sacrificial element in conventional treatment (surgery, radiation, chemotherapy)—the pain and suffering; the giving up of trophies in the guise of limbs, organs, glands, bits of skin and flesh—was what made it work. And how much the logic or apparent rationalism in the alternate methods was the effective element. In both, indecisiveness, imprecision, seem to prevail. Less of an admission of ignorance in the alternative methods perhaps than in the conventional ones, since the cancer surgeons and oncologists insist on sweeping up operations—as many as two or three—as insurance in case they are wrong or have overlooked something. But in both instances there is the frequent cry of "too late; if we had only known earlier, we could have got it all out." And for both there is the shadowy nature of the adversary. Where, exactly, does it come from? What governs its mysterious appearances and disappearances, its dawdling progress, its deadly rushes forward.

ONLY a couple of us look really sick, or even sick at all. I am not sure how sick I might appear to those who have never seen me before.

There is no question: the younger the person afflicted, the more the pathos and concern. Also, the younger the person, the more virulent, the quicker the advance of the disease.

WE went to Quaker meeting in the barn: big square space, padded pews on three sides of the square occupied by maybe sixty to seventy people. The healthy moving over for, accommodating the sick. I dozed off and dreamt I was in a Quaker meeting.

NEW arrivals.

Ralph R. and his wife. A small man with a beard. Eighteen months ago lymphoma diagnosed. Chemotherapy did the trick. Feels very lucky. "I have the cancer personality."

Beverly Y. Husband, a blacksmith, too ill to come. Cancer throughout the abdomen. Can't operate or radiate, and the chemotherapy is not working. Three small children. He is in great pain. Drugged. Hopeless. Finally tears. Real, gushing tears. The first.

Beverly's tears open up the meeting. Tom tells us he was given six months to live. Irene C. was given six months and refused treatment of any kind. It is now two years later.

> 7:30 P.M. Irene will help us with collage making at Brinton House. Each of us can try to express, through this medium, where we are going: "How do I see myself in the future?" We can display them afterwards; and, if we want to, say what we think is presented in them.
> End when we end!

A table full of bits and pieces, odds and ends. Old magazines, feathers, shells, scraps of paper, string, rags, scissors, buttons, paste, Scotch tape.

Out of this I make an idealized terrace of the big old hotel in Agrigento: looking out to sea, a green and white awning overhead, a triangular sail in the middle distance. An evocation of our honeymoon, where fear and hope seemed in perfect balance. We figured Elizabeth was conceived in our room with a view of the temples. The bed collapsed. Then on to Trapani, Segesta, Palermo, across the sea to Tunis, all the way to Mogador and back.

Ralph R.'s collage was scarcely more than three dots (seeds), a bent string glued to a white background.

I feel normal, healthy even. Not because so many here are worse off than I, though they may well be, but just because I now qualify for membership in an interesting, congenial group. I belong.

3.

10:00–11:30 A.M. Kitty will lead us in: *What are we learning?* Do we recognize our heightened consciousness? Accepting the challenge? Moving forward with Faith?

11:30–12:15. Visualization/worship sharing.

I unintentionally terminated the visualization exercise when I put us all aboard a balloon that rose from the courtyard of a crenellated castle where the last participant had barricaded us. A great striped balloon, I told them, was taking us away, with a handsome wicker basket, lifting off into a bright blue sky with fat white clouds, floating free, out and up and suddenly the sky is filled with other bright balloons just as free, swinging up and out into space. Far, far out. A perfect summer's day. After a few moments silence, during which the person whose turn was next obviously couldn't think of anything to do with an armada of rising scattering balloons, Howard burst into hearty song—"Allaloo, allaloo, allaloo"—and we broke for our farewell lunch.

New York City

1. I woke at two with an ocular migraine, a slight pain in the gut and a determination not to put in an appearance at the Du Pont ceremonies tonight, the climax of my work year, visible on the public broadcast system coast to coast. I don't intend to sit there like some sort of ritual object, saying nothing, a totem for all the world to observe and interpret. I've done little or nothing toward the event, having played the most elaborate sort of hooky for the last six months.

If I stay away, my absence could be ascribed to a temporary setback due to my therapy. Present, everyone can make his own diagnosis, which—under the circumstances of thinness and tiredness and God-knows-what expression I'll manage, of anxiety, boredom or just plain weariness—has to be negative.

A note from Mary Ellin left on the kitchen counter:

> Marvin, Here's what I'll do about the Du Ponts if you decide not to go. I'll go to the cocktail party, to greet friends and loved ones who've shown up in your honor, and faculty, and reassure everyone that you're not there for reasons of *temporary* depletion— then I'll come home to watch it on TV with you.

My decision made, you can make yours at five P.M.
Love, M.E.

I am not sure I want anyone reassured.

I have now seen Dr. C., who has told me that they are scaling
down the area of treatment to limit damage to the kidneys.
One kidney, apparently, they are willing to sacrifice. Also, he
tells me that without radiation the microscopic tumors would
have grown and spread in four to six months. So radiation isn't
simply insurance but a necessity. And I not only have to give
up half my stomach but half my kidneys as well. I think someone might have warned me of all this.

Furthermore, a defective kidney, they say, can lead to
hypertension. How does that fit in with my heart condition?
Dr. C. says, "Not at all." But I want someone else to say it.

I lay on the platform looking up into Big Mach's square maw,
which expands and contracts in response to some unseen button. There are planes inside planes and a source of light revealed as they part. What the devout Moslem seeks inside that
black cube in Mecca? The beatific vision? Not for me. I see the
enemy.

Dr. C. and Dr. I. say they have reduced the field to 65
percent of what it was before to protect one kidney. To hell,
apparently, with the other.

I called Dr. S. and asked him two questions: Is it imperative
that I sacrifice a kidney to this monster? And, if this will give

me hypertension, where does that leave my already defective heart? And, incidentally, while we're at it, why does Dr. C. talk as though radiation is not just insurance but therapy for a known condition—bits of lymphoma left lying about in my belly that without all those rads would inevitably grow and spread? Doesn't this indicate a less successful outcome to surgery than we originally assumed? I am indignant. I am more than indignant. I am incensed. All this fighting for my organs one by one is giving me a higher color than usual, which should be good for my appearance this evening at the DuPont Awards, both in the hall under those hard lights and out there, coast to coast on color TV.

So, out of orneriness, sudden resolve, defiance, I apparently have decided to go.

THE ceremony is over. I went to the prebroadcast party for the first time in half a dozen years. Usually I sit in a back room at Low Library guarding the celebrities' wraps, greeting the big names and answering their last-minute questions and complaints, hanging up their minks and Chesterfields, anything to avoid the mob scene across the rotunda amongst the priceless Chinese objets d'art. This time I met the rush head on, and it was rubber bumpers in all directions. If not love—neutrality. The subversion of all egos, mine most of all. An illusion, perhaps, but a happy one. Even the celebrities behaved themselves. Andy Rooney was wearing space shoes. Diane Sawyer glowed, soft, fuzzy like a peach. Linda Ellerbee was all hair and pep. Geraldo Rivera, David Brinkley, Susan Stamberg each on his or her good behavior.

I sat on the last chair on the dais. No searching looks.

No moist concern. Jim Morton came up to tell me his daughter Hilary is at home, suffering from the aftereffects of her next-to-last dose of chemotherapy—unpleasant, but still, the next to the last. He is going with a group of sixty likeminded people to Mt. Sinai to pray for peace. Moses' mountain, not the hospital.

On the way out, behind the coat racks, I ran into Terry Drinkwater, a winner for his miniseries on cancer—his own. I told him we had a CAT scan machine, a linear accelerator in common, congratulated him, for his cure, for his award, I don't know which.

"Until the next time," he said, and I'm not quite sure what that meant either.

MARTHA, who had promised me she would be there, without fail, hadn't shown.

I have a new drawing on my stomach. The lines are darker, thicker, another square drawn in blood.

2. Yesterday's *Times* carried an item about the city council of San Diego voting to replace their new state-of-the-art high-sodium street lamps, with a low-sodium model that would make the residents look like ghouls. An expensive choice, but the Palomar Observatory sixty miles to the north could again see the stars.

* * *

AT Church read the Old Testament lesson—Jacob and Esau. Not a nice story. Nothing to inspire me there. The San Diego City Council better.

I met Diana T. on Claremont, and she asked about my health. I told her I was in therapy.

"Radium?" she asked.

"No," I said. "A linear accelerator."

"What is that?" she asked.

"An atom smasher," I said.

She shook her head in wonder. Obviously, when Lionel was being treated, it wasn't offered as an option. Progress of a sort.

ON the bus going downtown, somewhere in the Nineties, a woman, long shabby coat, dirty hair, scuffed running shoes, sagging socks, not young, not that old, climbed aboard, first hoisting a large brown plastic trash bag and two outsized paper tote bags and then groaning on after, the whole process taking at least two missed lights. She gave her bags a seat and stood over them, and eventually, when the bus didn't fill up, sat down herself. In the seventies a gang of noisy twelve-year-olds piled on, and the conductor stopped one of them at the door. The kid shouted down the bus to his buddies for change. Before he could get a response, the bag lady reached into her pocket and produced a coin. He said, "Thank you," politely, desposited the coin, and rejoined his group.

Near Lincoln Center she descended, taking as long to get off as to get on. The new riders waiting to board looked at her with undisguised impatience and distaste. She smiled at them and dragged her burdens off down Broadway. A happy bag lady.

They are all happy says Mrs. L., our housekeeper. "They don't worry," she says. "They have given up worrying, or just given up." Mrs. L. gets up at 3:30 in the morning to clean a doctor's office before she comes to us. She told me about a friend of hers whose brother had a nervous breakdown fifty years ago after two months in the service, nowhere near combat; been in a VA hospital ever since, sound as a bug. We should be so healthy.

3. I have a feeling that they got the cancer, that it was all gone before they even began this radiation sequence.

I have never had the feeling that there was anything down there anyway. Certainly nothing seething, out of control. Even the lumps they cut out were simply my own imagining built on the fact that Dr. W. and the others told me something was there—no real conviction, nothing felt or seen. So the unreal has been removed by the unwitnessed, and the invisible is now attacking what is not left, and all I have to show for it is a scar down my belly. But whether it is gone or not, I have the uncomfortable feeling that if I have made one cancer I can make another. And now my stomach and my back, where I imagine my left kidney to be, don't feel so good.

I have written a note to Martha on a card I brought back from Assisi showing Giotto's version of the Flight into Egypt. "It is a journey, a search," I tell her, ignoring the flight. If you are the Holy Family or Francis, I suppose the journey and the flight are one and the same; the search continues whether you are flogging Brother Ass at Porziuncula or riding him into Jerusalem.

ON the Op Ed page of the *Times* a lady writes about "the synergistic causes of cancer," putting them all together—canvassing your environment and your diet for possible causes. Looking for others to blame besides yourself. In a world where the rules are forever changing, it seems a miracle that any one survives childhood.

But then there is the suspicion that every person, every thing, every event is unique, is an exception to the changing rules. We go blindly on, like moles, burrowing our own zigzagging tunnels until finally we reach the light.

4. Valentine's Day in the Tunnel. I met a baby in a crib with an IV being wheeled down the first-floor corridor. Below there was a six-year-old boy with half his hair shaved away coming off the machine and a group of half a dozen patients in wheelchairs and on stretchers waiting their turns. I told them at the desk that I had a rash, and Dr. C. saw me immediately. He found no reason for interrupting treatment, although the rash obviously comes from it. Now I am back waiting my turn. A radio audible in the background—some sort of busy dialogue.

I have never noticed the sign on the door to Big Mach. Three yellow triangles—Caution High Radiation Area. I sit beside a youngster with markings on his jaw; seven years old maybe, cereal-bowl haircut. I ask him which machine he is on.

He points to the twenty-two-million-volt one. Mine is only six.
Then the technician calls, "Hi, Matt, come on in."
The boy and I come out at the same time.

ON the subway I am overtaken by a senseless fear that
things will not change, that even if they manage a complete
cure, I will just do it all over again; that I won't have the
strength or desire to reverse the flow; that I will go right
back to attacking what is left of my poor stomach or some
other organ or my heart. That, obviously, is what heart attack means. Before I had always thought of its being attacked
from outside—a broken heart, a heartbreaker—but, of
course, that isn't it at all. There has to be someone on the
inside helping out. An inside job.

Something in me is reading what is going on—what has
been going on for years—as a death warrant. I know better.
But will I be able to untangle the signals in time.

At what point in this struggle, do you choose between life
and death? What—who—does the choosing, and is choosing
death ever the right choice? And are all these negative
thoughts—today, yesterday—not my fault but the fault of Big
Mach, 3800 rads. Too many doctors. Too many people sicker
than I. Death.

Gerald's death a decade ago: thousands of miles away,
Gerald lying in silence month after month, his red beard
white, his thin hands, thinner, more translucent still, an old
man, eighty or more, almost, but not quite a vegetable, saying
suddenly, out of nowhere, "It is taking rather a long time, isn't
it?" in that lovely Anglo-Irish accent of his that was such a
pleasure to hear no matter what he said. Even when he had
suggested to our horror that he, still in his fifties, might prefer

promotion from this middle world, release from his defective body, to the privilege of our eager company. He had had a long wait.

ANN H. called to say that Lord P. had died—some time last night or early this morning. He was seventy-six. Had a pacemaker. Somehow the heart got out of control. Very sudden. Someone else who seemed to know—gone.

5. The coffin, closed, was in front of the fireplace in what I assumed was the sitting room of the apartment in a big old duplex building in the East Sixties. There were four rows of chairs facing it. On the mantle was a clutter of found objects: shells, sand dollars, starfish, a chambered nautilus, a reproduction of a madonna and child, a Buddhist tanka, a French clock, a small figurine of a dervish, a picture of a man in old-fashioned clothes skating on a frozen pond.

I sat for twenty minutes with a dozen other people—two or three familiar faces. No family. No conversation. Not even a murmur. Silence. Palpable silence.

Close up, death seems less threatening, less disturbing. Something taken for granted. The funeral is tomorrow at St. Vincent Ferrar.

The priest was Lord P.'s friend. Whatever Lord P.'s religion—Anglican, Presbyterian, Russian Orthodox, none at all—it didn't seem to matter. The church would be full. They would sing "O God, Our Help in Ages Past" to an unfamiliar tune, read scripture as well as selections from Gurdjieff's *Beel-*

zebub, mill about in the sun outside the church when the service was over looking stunned.

A piece in *Life* on Tommy Thompson, who died at forty-nine of cancer of the liver. The piece pegged on the TV miniseries based on his novel *Celebrity* but really about the cancer. The author, *People Magazine* editor Richard Stolley, has a hard time making it all add up. Best-sellers, miniseries, death.

"Dick," Tommy said to his best friend after delivering his dire news—just a few weeks left to live—"you and I have already lived better, more exciting lives than most of the rest of the world." Not exciting enough, his pal seems to be replying, never exciting enough to justify the pain, the fear.

ETHEL Merman died today. An inappropriate thing for her to do.

6. Ran into Joan S. on the way back from Lord P.'s funeral. She knew about my cancer; had had a recurrence of her own—a second mastectomy. Bud, her husband, has had cancer for years. She said she was surprised, though, that I had gotten the dread disease: "What with your meditating and all. Why do you think you got it? Why hadn't the prayers prevented it?" These were good questions that no one besides myself has had the gall to ask so far. Maybe I sense the answer. My prayers have not been the kind that spare you illness. Survival prayers maybe, but survival at a cost.

* * *

"PRAYER is not asking for things—not even for the best things; it is going where they are." Gerald quoted in *The Choice Is Always Ours*, "an anthology of the religious way," one of the devotional books currently stacked on my bedside table. It was compiled by Lucille Nixon, last seen glowering by the sink in the kitchen at Trabuco, a devotee gone sour—not really—not for long. None of us stayed sour for long. That was Gerald's genius. To turn us off, brutally, or stand by while we turned ourselves off, and then, by remote control, across a continent, a couple of decades, to turn us on again. You never really shook Gerald.

IN the hospital elevator I met the little boy with the half-bald head, deeply shadowed eyes, a puffy, patient look. His mother was giving him his chit for his next round on Big Mach.

I have some dim understanding of why I might have cancer. Getting on the wrong track, trying to cross over, mashed in the crossing. But why him, who hasn't even had a chance to choose a track, to change his mind, to make a mistake? That of course is the crucial question. Why anyone? No easy explanations. No one around now that I would even consider asking.

Two kids already in the tunnel: two more six-year-olds.

MARY Ellin told me again last night that I was a good man. I didn't protest. Let her think so if she wants, if it makes her feel any better. It is certainly nothing that I feel or perceive.

Perhaps it is only perceptible to someone else and that perception is not transferrable. I suspect the moment you agree, the moment you feel good or see yourself as good, the illusion dissolves. I have seen that flickering reflection of goodness slipping over the horizon on those rare instances when I have achieved some act or thought of near generosity, of almost selflessness. And I have drawn back quickly, realizing that such squeaking self-approval is a portion of that reward we get here and not in heaven. I have witnessed what would appear to be goodness in others—in the nuns in the South Bronx, for instance, or an occasional nurse or doctor or clergyman—but I suspect they have no satisfaction in "being good," or, if they do, they are contrite about it, asking God, if they believe in him, to spare them such illusions.

Of course, I know how to appear to be good, to simulate goodness; that may be what M.E. is talking about. Not that it is easy to persist in such make-believe. If one pretended to be good long enough, steadily enough, one might actually become so. But there could be no vacations, recesses, coffee breaks from such playacting.

7. Jonathan Schell spoke at the cathedral this afternoon at a meeting for peace. Briefly. Said fear should be replaced by love—the only way to avoid nuclear destruction. So what else is new? But the fact that it isn't new doesn't make it any less true. Inside every cliché is the truth struggling to get out.

* * *

ORCHESTRA seats for *Cats*. Tedious and vulgar. All that money and effort squandered to no effect. There is no way to make clutter—in the head, in the heart, on stage—effective. That is what clutter is: insignificance, uselessness, meaningless detail. A cluttered life—even the most cluttered—death will set to rights. Like a magnet under a paper of iron filings.

8. Back to the cathedral for Sunday morning service. The prayer for the day was "O Lord, who hast taught us that all our doings without charity are nothing worth; send thy Holy Ghost and pour into our hearts that most excellent gift of charity, the very body of peace and of all virtues without which whosoever liveth is counted dead before Thee." A text for Jonathan Schell.

There was an ambulance in front of 35 Claremont. Mrs. B., on a stretcher, was being unloaded by the attendants and her grandson. She said something about having had an operation. I told her to get well. Is it more of the same? Could it have climbed all the way up to the eighth floor now.

An agenda has arrived from Jacksonville for the next meeting of the Du Pont Trustees. Nothing has changed except my stomach. Oz still says, "Wait and see." I am not so sure.

Listened to the Razoumovsky no. 1. A perfect piece of music. What does it say? That isn't the point. It is what it is. That is the advantage of music over words. Music can just be; doesn't have to mean. But what about the prayer at church yesterday.

9. At the tunnel I have suddenly become a familiar. Everyone knows me. The bearded technician calls me "Mr. B." Matthew—the kid with the cereal-bowl haircut—accepts me as one of them. There are now others who are new, strange, yet-to-be-assimilated—perhaps they never will be: three or four in the women's waiting room; a stretcher case; a handsome young man in a wheelchair pushed by his pretty girlfriend, or wife, or sister. I have seen him before. He sits there inert, no response, eyes open but not seeing. Whether it is despair or damage I can't tell.

Nothing new happens to me here now. I go in—press the square and the door to the back opens. I open the second door manually as I am supposed to. I no longer bother to take off my sweater and shirt and undershirt and put on a Johnny coat. I simply push them all up, off my belly, and climb onto the machine. I lie there like one of the luge riders in the winter Olympics rushing downhill in a tunnel of ice, only I am stationary, with the red streak falling down my chest, not quite centered. In a minute it is all over. I pull down my shirt, thank whoever the operator is, and leave, telling the woman at the desk I'll see her tomorrow. An old hand. An old stomach. Part of a stomach.

I called the American Cancer Society to find out if there was any increase in cancer deaths. A man tells me the incidence of cancer has gone from one in four to three in ten in the past ten or twenty years, he isn't quite sure which. No really reliable figures on cancer deaths are kept nationwide. Still, there are at least 450,000 cancer deaths annually. Heart disease is still a bigger killer: 700,000 deaths annually. But heart disease is declining as a cause of death. Cancer isn't. I don't know whether to believe him or not. He sounds as though he is making it up to get me off the phone.

I am back to visiting Mr. D. once a week in his single hotel room on upper Broadway.

This afternoon he enumerated the horrors of his life, saying all he wanted was love and the only person who had loved him was the rancher's wife in Texas who sent him out into the world with two dollars and a bandana on a stick as a young orphan boy—after her husband had brutalized him. He also told me the story of his tic douloureux—the agony, the treatment—and his marriage to a successful woman in show business who proposed to him. A marriage of convenience it turned out to be—her convenience. She had a boyfriend in Sing Sing who arrived one evening with a revolver and told him to get out and stay out, marriage or not. "If I ever see you again, I'll kill you." Mr. D. got out. As for his teeth and glasses, still more delays. His urinary tract is bothering him again, his back. He doesn't eat or sleep.

I left him a biography of Helen Morgan, whom he had known in the old days. "A great talent," he said. "A mess. Her own worst enemy."

10. In the midst of prayers this A.M., floating up through all the distractions, was Mildred Bailey's sweet, reedy voice and the words "the captive maid is mute." Scrabbling back into my past I finally located the words, the terminal line from hers and Red Norvo's recording of "From the Land of the Sky Blue Water," last heard on the old phonograph in my attic room in Des Moines, in 1947, lying on great Uncle Peter's four-poster bed. Billie Holiday's "Travellin' Light," Ivy Anderson's "I've Got It Bad," Marion Harris's "I Can't Get the One I Want." ("Those I get I don't want. Babies I long for, Never go strong for meeee.")

That took care of prayers.

A rousing passage from Philippians at service this morning: "Brethren, I count not myself to have apprehended; but this one thing I do, forgetting those things which are behind, and reaching forth unto those things which are before, I press toward the mark for the prize of the high calling of God. . . ."

Pam tells me Hilary is finished with chemotherapy but doesn't know what comes next. From here on out there is no vocabulary.

AFTER an afternoon of runny bowels and bleak thoughts I was cheered by Irving, who came into the bedroom and showed me his latest work of art. A lot of diddly little squares I have seen him working on for weeks at his bench in the living room in front of the TV—"The Honeymooners," the "Late Night Movie." Suddenly, he has cut it up and put it back together. There it is moving around within itself, making wonderful sense.

11. I woke this A.M. with a bad taste in my mouth, light-headed in a heavy way—heavy in the limbs. Prayers. Still felt lousy.

Now I am in the tunnel waiting for Dr. I. to make sure

it is all right to go on the machine. My forearms ache. I feel breathless like I have been walking uphill. I want to make sure it isn't my heart, that the machine isn't doing something it shouldn't be. The technician agrees. I should wait.

I leave and go downtown to My cardiologist's office. Dr. C. and Dr. I. concurred. The symptoms may not be severe, but they are obviously provocative.

Miles's first reaction was to clap me into the cardiac care unit for observation. Then he decided an office exam would do as well. Now I have had a cardiogram, a blood test, a physical. I have been confined to quarters for the weekend. I am to take double doses of Cardizem and keep Demerol on hand in case of an emergency. He thinks it is angina, although there are no chest pains. No one has mentioned angina before. Grandmother Barrett died of angina. Overnight, or so at least it seemed to me at eight. The fatal sickness brought on by grief at Eddy's death. The crime compounded.

THE little boy with no immune system died in his bubble out in Texas yesterday after declaring his willingness "to go home" and winking at the doctor.

12. I have now completed my first twenty-four hours in the back bedroom. To judge by the bright wall opposite reflecting the sun, it is a fine day out. Still, I do not feel well enough to resent my immobility. I have improved my time by listening to the Brahms First, with its huge engine grinding away inside it, moving the great slithery blocks of sound back and forth.

Then I began Solzhenitsyn's *The Cancer Ward* which, in its first few pages, has given me more of a sense of common cause in the dire meaning—the desperation of our lot—than I have had so far in my various hospitals or certainly among the hopeful people at Pendle Hill; the possibility that we all may be slipping down, rather than climbing up, whatever incline we are on—the authentic sense of tilt.

Even in the tunnel surrounded by people in obviously desperate shape—on stretchers, in wheelchairs, ambulatory; babies, old men and women wasted, scabbed by their disease—I don't feel that wobble, that communion of desperation. The book makes it quite clear. Makes the disease real, inside and out. My disease. His disease. Their disease. Our disease.

MARY Ellin just killed a cockroach on the wall behind my pillow. I thought I saw something climbing across the blue sweater Elizabeth knit me, but I attributed it to faulty vision. We don't have cockroaches in the bedroom. In the kitchen, sometimes in the bathroom, but never in the bedroom. "Perhaps it is my condition that attracts them," I said to Mary Ellin when she made some comment about the grubbiness of life. "Besides," I said, "it is just part of the richness and variety. The cockroach, squashed, will come back in a higher form. Ahimsa."

13. I wake at five. My mouth tastes better, but I am still weak and queasy and my bowels are watery. I realize I don't know what to do; what next. Should I say categorically, no more radiation? Has this latest episode justified such a course, or would I be malingering? Is malingering possible in the midst of all this therapeutic activity? Or must I go on until the cure is finished? But when is it finished? There seems to be a vagueness about the number of rads required. I am over 3,500 now. Different people have different limits and different levels of tolerance, I have been told. Have they exceeded mine? Should I have refused treatment to begin with like my friends at Pendle Hill? Should I have saved my stomach and risked my life? Haven't I been risking it all along?

Why, at this point, are all these questions occurring to me?

MEANWHILE life goes on.

Today I have talked to all the children. Elizabeth reports Sasha is coming along on the piece commissioned by the Berkeley Symphony. He and the conductor had dinner night before last to discuss it. Mary Ellin Jr. on top of a full schedule at *Family Weekly* is working on a piece on agoraphobia for *Woman's Day* to make some extra money. Katherine is trying to decide whether she should come back from Rome two weeks early, give up the classics to take a job at *Cosmopolitan.* Irving is going downtown to interview for a job at the Museum of Modern Art and get himself a new raincoat, our valentine present to him.

Some people, as they grow old and sick, seem to look at their children with increasing fear and distaste, perceiving them as invaders, intruders, rather than comforters; not as their chance at immortality, but as the instruments of their mortality—the inheritors, the ones who are going to get it all (the world, their place in it) when they are gone and therefore, one way or another, must be responsible for their going. If they avoid them, if they give them no token of their love, they may forestall the fateful day.

So far, thank God, my children don't frighten me. Nor can I imagine this ever happening. They are friends, companions, whom I love and find comfort in. Besides I don't think of them as my sole chance for immortality. We all, young and old, have an equal shot at that, a shot that can't miss the target.

14. My weekend confinement is over. The arm symptoms have not recurred. Miles has told me to go back to my schedule. So despite my fantasies of being taken off the machine, I am in line, waiting my turn.

HEAVY rain, driving easterly winds, the *Times* says. Miserable, cold, impossible to keep an umbrella up. For the first time in four weeks I have forgotten my glasses and it is a waiting day. Twenty minutes early for my nine o'clock appointment. The homeless man is here already in his Johnny coat, looking bad. The man from Queens says the worst thing about all this—the cancer, the radiation therapy—is the subway ride in from the Island. There were three abandoned umbrellas on the pavement outside the entrance to Babies Hospital. I barely got mine closed.

*　*　*

BACK under Big Mach. Another 180 rads. B. says maybe Thursday will be my last day. She tells me there is a lot of cement and maybe some lead in the ceiling I am staring at. And above that a garden. Not a good place to take a walk, although the flowers don't seem to mind. She points to the African violets under the lavender light.

There is a new square on my stomach. They have reduced the field by several centimeters, thus eliminating the heart completely.

I label everyone in the tunnel—the old-timers like myself: the Hispanic lady, the homeless one, the man in loafers, the man from Queens, the kid with the cereal-bowl haircut. How am I labeled? The tall thin one? I didn't use to be thin. Even when I was, people thought of me as chubby, round-faced. Now I am haggard. The white-haired man in the outdoor jacket, the gray astrakhan hat, the scuffed Frye boots.

Tomorrow, ostensibly, this sequence which began last July will be complete. And then, if I choose, life will proceed, deeper and richer, more troubled and tormented—however I want it—than ever. Except perhaps for a little clicking in the background—life's metronome, life's clockwork bomb—reminding me of time if I am so fortunate as to forget it, or stop it, or rise above it, out of it, like Saint Joseph of Copertino through the chapel ceiling, past all those lovely pictures of Saint Martin of Tours, out through the roof and into another dimension where there is no need to move at all. A pause, like one in making love, that you rise into.

My stomach bothers me. The smashed atoms seem to be getting to me as they haven't before.

I itch. My shoulders and my legs. The mutilated atoms perhaps are protesting.

I went to the India Travel Office and got literature for my trip to Darjeeling and Benares. I intend to go, whatever the altitude. Two weeks of staring at the Himalayas from the veranda of the Windamere.

March

15. My stomach woke me for the first time really since I began radiation. Not from pain—just presence. And inside of nothing, a petrified, clarified burp. And that nasty taste, or lack of taste, in the mouth. Again the "nothing there" syndrome. The absent sensation.

THERE are moments when to replace a light bulb seems too much of a challenge. Of course, the light bulb in the kitchen ceiling is not all that easy to replace. You have to stand on the counter, remove the white translucent globe, three screws to unset and set. A balancing act when one's balance is very uncertain.

MY last wait.

The man from Queens tells me about a new laser treatment for cancer he read about in the *National Geographic.*

The little thin boy just walked by with his mother.

A 12 year old girl in pink pants and a flat white beret balanced on top of her head.

A tall man in a chartreuse hat with a cane.

A young woman in a wheel chair with a shower cap on her head.

The hairless business man in pin stripes and loafers looks better, more alert.

Everyone is here to see me off.

The homeless man in checked pants, plaid shirt, purple sweater—leather jacket—indelible lines running down both sides of his neck.

A tiny girl in a blue corduroy pinafore holding a bottle—dutch bob.

Man in work clothes, jeans, blue canvas galoshes with cream rubber soles, flap cap, gray hair.

Middle aged man in grey worsted suit with ruined face sits reading *Newsweek*. A blonde in a black pants suit with a wolf collar.

When I get up from the slab and say good-bye, B., the technician, says she hopes never to see me again.

Dr. C. says I have done very well. No vomiting, no dysentery. At least not enough to make special pills worthwhile. Good basic condition. Maybe in a month, I'll be back to normal.

At the outer desk I sign up for an appointment three months from now. A fragile young woman comes off the elevator, a wraith, shoulders drooping, her handbag hanging around her neck, weighing her down.

Waiting behind me is a young man, maybe twenty, missing an arm and all his hair, signing up for radiation. The chemo, the surgery haven't been enough.

I leave.

* * *

TO celebrate, we went to dinner and Sam Shepard's *Fools for Love* with Oz and Inger. Everyone loved dinner, hated the play, except for me. The dinner I could take or leave; the play was a heluva lot better than *Cats,* I said.

The violently slammed door was a recurrent motif throughout the evening. On stage, a hundred, two hundred slammed doors. Slammed hard. A farce without the fun. The cab we got home had an uncatchable rear door. For eight blocks I tried to get it properly shut—a couple of dozen unsuccessful slams. Finally the driver went back to the garage, leaving us on a street corner waiting for another ride.

The door to the apartment slammed and locked against all intruders.

It was a day and a night of slamming doors.

Now, perhaps, I can begin to get well.

IV.

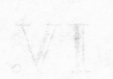

St. Luke's

1. The oxygen tube makes me think I have my glasses on. The defunct TV set reflects a constellation on its screen, little pinpoints of light from the monitor opposite, a Cassiopeia of sorts. Four bags are suspended from the ceiling. They have some connection with me but I can't make it out. There are four readings. Three look serious. One meaningless. I am not sure which is which. There is a huge window slatted with a venetian blind. I have no idea what is behind it. A gay canvas curtain, bright stripes, protects me from the big room.

Now that my legs are shaking, they don't itch so much.

In the next cubicle is a young woman with a respirator that changes its rhythm and sound periodically. The two nurses talk to her. The patient doesn't answer back. At least, I can't hear her.

THERE were three policemen in the patrol car. The one in the back seat asked me what made me so sure I was having a heart attack. Very polite, I said I had had one before and knew what it was like. Mary Ellin, less polite, told them to step on it. Finally they turned on their flashing light and made that nasty whooshing noise they can make under the revolving blue and drove fast down Broadway to 112th Street, then left toward the cathedral, another sharp left at the broad shallow steps with the scaffolding climbing up one end, a squealing right, and into the emergency bay.

A roomful of people waiting. They could have been sitting just so since the last time I was there. And the time before that. The same young man slumped across his chair, hand over eyes. The students giggling. The bag lady staring at the clock on the wall. The man with the bandaged eye.

At the desk they were in no hurry. Rustled some papers. Asked questions. Looked at me with narrowed eyes. Finally they let us in.

I was in the same alcove I had been in last July when the symptoms they thought were heart-related in the end signaled cancer. The nurse flapped the curtain shut. Out there it was all hustle. The sense of people sicker, more needful than I. After a long wait an orderly came to take me upstairs.

THEY tell me that I was dead sometime this afternoon. Not all that dead. With a little effort—a blow to the chest, a few electric shocks, a team of six working at it—they were able to bring me back to life. Sort of dead.

This is the way I recall it. A green slope: not slippery, not furry—like sealskin—irregular, but not bumpy, slipping but not grabbing to hold on. No panic—nothing disagreeable— the green very bright, like new grass. Not shale, no precipice. No one on the bank above cheering me on. Me alone. I am doing as I should. Letting go. Relaxed. Out of the tunnel—not into it. Lots of light but not blinding. Like the shoot-the-chutes at Riverview Park in Des Moines—one downward plunge, the same quick quiet slide, the cushion of water at the bottom. No charge. Uncle Will Galbraith, an old man with a game leg who lived in a fleabag hotel off Mulberry Street and came to family dinners, took the tickets. No question of turning back, getting off. Then all of a sudden the delicious ride is over, the friendly green blinks out. The rattling and shaking, the dull roar, the low murmuring voices are back. I have returned.

I have no memory of saying, "Doctor," although apparently I did when I began to slip, as though I wanted someone to stop me. Not out of terror, resistance to what was coming. Still, not ready to go all the way. So I am back. Spinning. Uncertain. My legs shaking.

The heart was obviously jealous of all the attention my cancerous stomach had been getting. The surgery. The radiation. Forty-five hundred rads in not so easy doses. Half a stomach. Half a heart. Eat less—love more. A new admonition.

Falstaff when he was dying babbled of green fields.

IT happened on Sunday, two days after the night of the slamming doors.

At church, standing for hymns, for prayers, the Creed, I could hardly hold my overcoat up. During Communion, and then standing in line to greet the dean and the preacher of the day, the coffee hour, I thought I'd sink under my own weight. Somehow I got down the steps, up Amsterdam, across College Walk, eight blocks. Back home I took a call from Jean S., who asked how I was feeling now that the radiation was all over. I told her just fine—the ultimate, perhaps the penultimate lie—hung up, and had a heart attack. Mary Ellin went for a taxi; no nonsense about waiting an hour and a half for an ambulance this time. I occupied myself with the nitroglycerine bottle. With a heroic effort I got through the paper seal stretched across the top, dug the cotton out, and then, slowly, carefully shook out two very small pills to lay under my tongue.

There were no cabs. Mary Ellin found the patrol car with its three skeptical occupants sipping coffee and reading the *News* parked alongside Chock Full o'Nuts at 116th and Broadway.

I remember being dead once before: on the eve of Halloween fifty-nine years ago. A sledding accident. A boulder that had been at the bottom of the hill since the Pleistocene waiting for me. Dr. Langdon brought me back. No blow to the chest. No defibrillators. Whatever the magic was in 1925 administered in the nick of time. There were the same voices fifty-nine years ago. Above me, around me. The circle of heads. The murmuring quiet busyness. It wasn't me fighting for my life or giving up. It was everyone out there making the effort, pulling me back, a five-year-old with all his life before him. They did the same for Mother, twenty years ago, all bent over her bed. Trying, but not succeeding. The nun saying, "No. Not in there." But I had already seen—that it was hopeless. It was what they must have done with Eddie—too late. Why me? Pulled back twice—once early, once late—for what? Not counting all those times death just missed me in between: those I know about—the Aleutians, the Solomons, the Ryukyus—and those I don't know. The debt never called in. The others going on.

I can remember Dr. Langdon sitting in a Morris chair by

---

a bright window being told, "This is the boy whose life you saved." Unable to reply, he just looked at me, the pretty, frightened seven-year-old, scrubbed, in his best knickers, being pushed forward by his grateful mother for one last look. The life-giver was dying himself.

It was the next year I killed Eddie.

A day of drowsing. After the CBS Evening News I went to sleep in earnest. Dreamt. One dream from 7:30 P.M. to 5 A.M. Three interruptions by nurses. Pills, injections. Back to the dream. The remarkable thing was that I had dreamed the same dream before—the same unusual length, the same details. I recognized it in all its particulars and yet, awakened, I retained none of them. Still, I plunged back into it following each interruption, taking it up exactly where I left off. How long ago it was when I last had this dream, where, under what circumstances, I don't know. But there it was—vast, detached, pleasant, holding my interest firmly, irretrievable until the next time. All of a piece. Nothing dramatic to break it off. Why did I ever leave it?

I don't think about my cancer anymore except to think I am not thinking about it. It is wiped out. Not that this heart attack has replaced it. It hasn't. I just don't think about much of anything. Maybe it is the morphine or the Valium or God.

THE machines are wonderful. Huge in my modest cubicle. Machine number one: a black shiny garbage bin that does three-dimensional cardiograms. It looks like something an adolescent stage manager might dream up for a high school science fiction fantasy. The operator is as outlandish as the machine: a huge, red-headed woman, perhaps 350 pounds, who sits at the console—after having strapped me to it—creating elegant figures on the moving paper. I know her from my former life. She has three children, a Vietnamese husband, lives in Jersey. Or is that someone else?

Machine number two: white, with projecting arms. The cubicle can barely accommodate it. It is, I am told, an isotope machine. It has a heterogeneous elegance about it, articulated tubes connecting one geometric part to the next. To participate in its particular game one has radium injected in one's neck artery; then round objects begin to appear on a dark screen, shimmering, then resolving into the shapes of sherbet on hot lineoleum. I have no idea how to read them. It isn't considered important that I should.

I have been in the cardiac care unit now for almost a week, in my little cubicle. Irving came yesterday with a small picture to dress it up: a collage of collars, snakes eating their own tails, spirochetes in gentle colors.

THE night sounds: the pounding to clear someone's chest, the voices at the control desk with its rank of monitors, the clanging of the bell when a new patient arrives or there is an emergency on the floor requiring team effort . . . at once. An intense huddle of young doctors and nurses. A week ago the bells were clanging and the huddle was for me.

✻   ✻   ✻

WE in the cubicles facing the nurses' station are the elite, the alarmingly, dangerously sick. Down the hall beyond the monitors are the convalescents, shuffling about in their striped robes and paper slippers, gray in the face but mending.

My world for a week now. My room. Not a room really, since one wall is the striped curtain strung two feet from the ceiling and two feet short of the floor.

In the center—me, in my electric bed. Above is control central with its eternal blue-green wobbly line. The wobble represents me—alive. A small flashing yellow light, a number (my pulse), two pale-yellow squares, meaning unknown, and a whole wall of buttons, switches, plugs, etc. Next to it, toward the window, some sort of console with a needle indicator is plugged into a red wall outlet with two odd gray-and-red, vaguely sexual (doglike) projections. It seems inert. At least the needle doesn't move.

On the rolling bed table: the blue device with the tiny Ping-Pong ball to increase my breathing capacity, seven plastic cups, the ice-water container, a box of tissues, my glasses case, and a stack of books. At the top Waugh's *Decline and Fall* at the bottom George Herbert's *Poems,* somewhere in between Merton's *Asian Journals,* Olivia Manning's Balkan trilogy, a couple of murder mysteries.

The blue pills are beta blockers, the pale-green are Cardizem, the bright-orange ones are for chest pain. Plenty of nitroglycerine. If they dropped me I'd blow the place up.

Mary Ellin tells me that now in the next cubicle an enormously fat man is being visited by his enormously fat wife and three enormously fat children. She doesn't know how they all fit in.

* * *

I have been moved beyond the monitors. My roommate is the fat man from the adjacent cubicle. He has the window bed and the color TV with the ballgame on.

In my bathrobe and slippers I am wandering about, staring back at the row of cubicles where I, as one of the really desperate cases, used to be. I can see a bandaged hand in one alcove which seems to motion to me. At the far end an old woman sits up in her bed noticing no one. And in the cubicle next to her is a body with two of what appear to be knives stuck in its exposed belly.

It is 5 A.M., and most, if not all, of the Cardiac Care Unit, seems to be asleep. My roommate is snoring peacefully, or almost peacefully, an occasional snarl interrupting the regular rhythm.

I have been lying awake since four, thinking.

I hit some sort of barrier Sunday before last, head on, and then, after the green sliding—the fragmentation—life as I have been living it resumed, but with a difference. And now it was Ash Wednesday, and I was being wheeled to chapel and what seemed to be the certainty of tears during the Our Father—nothing more familiar, nothing stranger—and then the chaplain making the smudge in the middle of my forehead, and returning me to quarters.

THE fat man has put on a bright-red running suit, packed his dufflebag, and left for the other side of the hospital.

Now it is just me, my flowers and the TV set, and a clear view of the window. Space—all the space I need.

*　*　*

A bright-blue wheelchair has come to take me back to where
I used to be in Scrymser Pavilion last July. And last September.
For the moment there is no one in the second bed. Next door
the loggia with its summer furniture, its big windows facing
east and west, is cold and deserted.

Don't forget this scene.

Miles, my longtime support, is standing by the window—
north, streaming light—and I am beside him. He has just done
one of those things he does: tapped my chest, looked at that
vein that runs behind my ear while he jabs the side of his hand
into my belly. On the table beside the bed is a spectacular
pyramid of orchids from my parents-in-law and Irving's congregation of shimmering rings. On the sill are the tulips from
Jean S., growing taller, more translucently yellow by the hour.
I am standing—not so straight as I might, but straight
enough—in my favorite dark green silk Sulka wrapper, beautifully cut, very smart, I think, not knowing that the right elbow
is out and my pajamas showing through. And opposite us—
Miles, me, Mary Ellin, the flowers, the window, Irving's visionary rectangle—are four young doctors—two men, two
women—half my age.

And suddenly Miles, with his look of incredible smooth-
ness—not quite smooth, smooth with a moss of intelligence,
of thoughtfulness—makes a tight, emphatic gesture in my direction and says simply: "Dead." But he wasn't saying, "This
was dead and look at him now, poor object that he is." I
have at least made an effort—shaved, combed my hair, put
on slippers and pajamas and my favorite wrapper—for this
encounter.

"Dead." And although I don't know quite what he is
saying to those young people starting out on their lifetimes of

saving lives, or to himself, a man at the peak of his career, his successes still outnumbering his failures two to one, if anything he does can be called a failure, I know what he was saying to me. I was dead—dead. The blue-green line was flat—without a wobble. I was at the bottom of the silky, limpid falls, lying there, not exactly senseless, nor certainly unconscious, but waiting, wondering, what next? And now I am alive again—for how long, who knows?—alive with half a stomach and God knows how many truant cells deciding, now that Big Mach is no longer there, which mischievous way they'll go next—half a stomach, and a notional, scatty heart.

"Dead," Miles says again and shoots out his elegant, precise hand with its spotless nails, looks at us all—Mary Ellin in her smart skirt and sweater, the young doctors in their smocks with their clipboards and stethoscopes and their sensible shoes—with an expression of triumph, puzzlement. "Dead," he says—flat, emphatic—and he means only "Alive."

THE day before he died Rabbi Shneur Zalman asked his grandson, "Is the ceiling still there?" When the boy said nothing, the Rabbi continued, in a voice quivering with joy, "I can see no ceiling or walls. I can only see the life of everything, and God creating everything and making everything live."

KATHERINE'S birthday. I am alone on the loggia before dawn. The table trays are full of cigarette butts and a plastic cup or two. The lamps on Morningside Heights are on, lighting up the dirty snow and leafless trees. Four brutal spots shine across Harlem from La Guardia. Yankee Stadium is dark, but you can see the pale silhouette of Mount Sinai, a shadow behind a shadow, down the park. There are vagrant lights here and there on the surface of Harlem and on the river beyond. It is too cold to open the French doors and go out onto the porch to see what is visible farther south or farther north.

A black man in a spotless white suit and shoes comes in, lights a cigarette. We nod. He moves on.

As I walk through this wing everything seems twice as old as six months ago, comatose, not likely to awake. Two or three nurses drift down the empty hall, or sit quietly reading at their desks in the blind corridor across from my room.

Back in Cardiac Care, where I was a week ago, all night the light was bright and sharp, the nurses and doctors young and busy, the machines new, vigilant.

Now I hear an old woman crying over and over again somewhere out there in her own dark room. "Please put it down." Again and again. After ten minutes the screaming subsides, then resumes, more subdued. Something out of control, unreachable by human hand or chemical substance or machine, is there in the darkness, now laughing, now sobbing.

MERTON writes about the marginal man, the monk, the displaced person, the prisoner, those who live in the presence of death and go beyond it to become "witnesses to life." Why does he leave the other experts off his list—the old, the desperately ill?

JIM Morton came in last night, fresh from the Holy Land, and gave me a piece of rose-colored stone from the top of Mount Sinai which he had picked up at dawn on Ash Wednesday. It is in the pocket of my dressing gown. Hilary is fine. Out looking for a job. They all hope to see me back at the Thursday morning service very soon. Things move as always for Jim. Things move.

BACK in my room it is six o'clock, and after a series of hilarious, high-spirited dreams—good-natured, affectionate—involving people I'd never seen before, I wake to hear the little man in the next bed with the double-bypass and valve transplant—whose wife died of emphysema nine months ago (surgery couldn't help her)—breathing hard, long breaths.

I am lying, not in a puddle of blood, or water, or a dirt-lined hole, but in that lukewarm funny soup that God brewed a billion years ago, waiting to be born. Again.

The sun is coming up.